RICHARD ASKWITH

Richard Askwith has been a journalist for over 40 years. He has written six previous books, including his modern classic on fell running, *Feet in the Clouds*, which won the Best New Writer category at the British Sports Book Awards and was shortlisted for the William Hill and Boardman Tasker prizes, and he is now one of the UK's most celebrated writers on running. *Running Free* was shortlisted for the Thwaites-Wainwright Prize, and his evocative biography of Emil Zátopek, *Today We Die A Little*, was shortlisted in the Cross Sports Book Awards. His most recent book, *Unbreakable: the Countess, the Nazis and the World's Most Dangerous Horse Race*, won Biography of the Year at the Telegraph Sports Book Awards in 2020.

RICHARD ASKWITH

The Race Against Time

Adventures in Late-Life Running

VINTAGE

1 3 5 7 9 10 8 6 4 2

Vintage is part of the Penguin Random House group of companies
whose addresses can be found at global.penguinrandomhouse.com

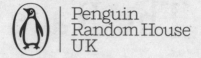

Penguin
Random House
UK

First published in Vintage in 2024
First published in hardback by Yellow Jersey in 2023

Copyright © Richard Askwith 2023

Richard Askwith has asserted his right to be identified as the author of this
Work in accordance with the Copyright, Designs and Patents Act 1988

penguin.co.uk/vintage

Printed and bound in Great Britain by Clays Ltd, Elcograf S.p.A.

The authorised representative in the EEA is Penguin Random House
Ireland, Morrison Chambers, 32 Nassau Street, Dublin D02 YH68

A CIP catalogue record for this book is available from the British Library

ISBN 9781529112368

Penguin Random House is committed to a sustainable future
for our business, our readers and our planet. This book is made
from Forest Stewardship Council® certified paper.

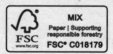

Contents

1

Scree slope

I had eaten too much breakfast, as easily happens when I visit the Lake District. My thighs and calves were trembling from the unaccustomed miles of climbing, and the June morning felt sticky. Even on the high fells, there didn't seem to be enough oxygen in the air, and what there was tasted of Cumberland sausage.

The ground began to level out near the summit of Bow-fell, and we roused ourselves into another determinedly upbeat jog. I hope that, had you seen us, you would have recognised us as fell-runners, but at that speed you can't be sure. We picked our way fussily through the sharp-edged rocks, barely gaining ground on the walkers up ahead. In our minds, however, we were running.

Twenty-five years earlier, though: you should have seen us then. We'd barely have slowed down for a boulder field like this; and if we did it was only to gather our energies for the next breakneck descent. We ran on these Cumbrian fells so often we could read the rocks, picking out safe footholds without conscious thought. We ran so confidently you could almost mistake us for locals. We could keep going for hours, too; all day if necessary. Often, we did.

Now, however . . . Well, we weren't racing. We weren't running against the clock. We were just out to enjoy a few hours on a much-loved route, making the most of the scenery and each other's company and proving to ourselves that we could still do it. The only problem was: I wasn't sure that we could.

The four of us running were the lucky ones: the ones who had kept in shape. The original plan for the weekend had been to get the whole team back together: getting on for twenty keen runners, all southerners, who back in the 1990s had devoted implausibly large amounts of energy and free time to conquering the challenges of the fells. But messy middle-aged reality kept thwarting us. There were overseas work commitments; a double hip replacement; an unanticipated mid-life family; illnesses and bereavements. We had first pencilled in a date two years earlier, then postponed it so that our guiding spirit could receive urgent cancer treatment. Twelve months later, coronavirus had locked us down; and now we were all two years older. We had barely noticed where the time had gone.

A dozen of the team had eventually made it up to Borrowdale, along with some long-suffering partners. If we had waited for everyone to be fit and available it would never have happened. As it was, eight of the notional runners who did join us declared themselves no longer fit for anything more arduous than hiking. It didn't matter. The joy of the weekend came from the group walks and the fell-side picnic and the long evenings of hilarious, beer-lubricated reminiscence; and the half-forgotten beauty of the mountains on two perfect June days; and the fact that we were finally old enough to admit, sheepishly, that we were quite fond of one another.

But the running: that was the tricky bit. I was in my

early sixties; Charles, Sarah and Titch were in their mid-fifties. Barring interruptions for injuries (rather frequent, in my case), we had barely changed our running habits since the old days, apart from a natural dialling-down of the obsessive intensity. We thought of ourselves as fit, but it was a long time since we had tested ourselves against the fells, and today's test was turning out to be unexpectedly tough.

Maybe the mountains had grown. Maybe the Earth's gravitational pull was stronger than before. Or perhaps there was something wrong with my legs. My muscles felt not just weak but empty. (Should I have had *more* for breakfast?) The day was still young, though, and we had miles of our planned circuit still ahead of us. So we banished negative thoughts and kept going, as you tend to do once the fell-running habit is in your blood. We worked our way briskly along the Scafell massif, via Esk Pike and Great End, before veering round and up towards Scafell Pike; and most of the time the sheer joy of being so high up on a clear morning distracted us from our physical difficulties. I felt knackered but also breathtakingly free: closer to the shining sky than to my grey worries below. The overwhelming continuity of the fells – vast and solid as they had been since before there were any human eyes to marvel at them – encouraged a strange sense of timelessness. At moments I even forgot that life had changed us, and imagined that we were still the thoughtless, careless, footloose young people we had all once been, twenty-five years earlier.

But you cannot ignore your body's protests for ever. My muscles were still empty and faltering, and as we worked our way up towards the summit of Scafell Pike I repeatedly stumbled. Or rather: I felt the crumbling path

3

slip and scatter beneath my feet. I seemed to be heavier than the other three as well as weaker. At any rate, I was finding things harder, and every now and then I had to put on a spurt to catch up. But those loose stones really weren't helping.

I thought back to all the times I had powered up this path in the past. The idea of finding it difficult offended me, so I blocked the discomfort from my mind. Onward and upward. Tiredness is for tourists.

We reached the summit, later than I had hoped, but eventually, even so. We marvelled at the clarity of the views. We talked about how lucky we were to be here: to have, still, the strength and the freedom to speed up to the highest point in England under our own steam, because we wanted to; and to know the best routes from one peak to the next; and to have legs that were capable (I hoped) of following them. And I thought: imagine not being able to do this any more; or, worse, imagine no longer being able to enjoy any kind of running at all. Be grateful, I told myself; and I was.

Then we headed off towards Great Gable, briefly enjoying the thought that whatever came next had to be downhill; and soon we were scrambling down the great, grey scar of scree slope on Scafell Pike's north-west side, feeling rather pleased with ourselves.

I used to love this descent: fast, yielding, a little crazy, but easier than it looks, if you go for it. This time, though, I kept stumbling. My feet seemed fractionally slower than they used to be – slower to respond to signals from my brain – and the resulting missteps twice prompted spasms of cramp in my calves. Distracted, I scrambled too far down the hill and then had to battle my way back up to the solid path of the Corridor Route. I was falling behind my friends again; so, again, I tried to power my way upwards. But the harder I pushed, the faster the loose rocks slipped from beneath me and rumbled downwards.

At one point, I felt a flash of fear. If I ended up in too big a landslide, in an unlucky direction, I could imagine slipping backwards uncontrollably towards a nasty drop. Then I paused, edged sideways, worked my way up more cautiously; and before too long I was back on the path, a little more shaky-legged than before but still just about jogging.

At Sty Head we paused. Our non-running friends had hiked up for a picnic, so we joined them for a while. Then, rested but not much refreshed, we set off again up Great Gable, on the dry, stone steps, with the afternoon sun (as often happens here) blazing too hot for comfort. I distracted myself with memories from our younger days, in which fell-running played such a big and life-enhancing part that I ended up devoting my first ever book, *Feet in the Clouds*, to the subject. My adult life might have taken a very different course had fell-running not awakened my dreams and my daring; and I have never quite been able to express my full gratitude to the friends who facilitated that awakening.

One of those mentors, Charlie (not the same as Charles), was still enjoying the picnic back at Sty Head. Repeated bouts of gruelling chemotherapy had left him temporarily unable to do more than labour uphill at a slow plod, gasping for breath. But he did so with the same cheerful, patient, understated, pig-headed courage that had made him such a formidable fell-runner half a lifetime earlier, and my thoughts about his unbreakable spirit seemed to strengthen my resolve too. If he could, I should. No matter how interminable the steep climb seemed, I would not let Great Gable defeat me.

The summit came, as summits do, after what felt like an hour or more. We hobbled gratefully down the steep, bouldery path on the far side, and then, some time later, headed as fast as we could up the crumbling track from Windy Gap, up towards Green Gable. I noticed that I had fallen behind again, so I put on another spurt, and, once again, my feet slipped crazily on the loose, pink stones. I began to feel sorry for myself – absurdly, in the general circumstances – and wondered why these gravitational mishaps kept happening to me. They never did in the past – or had I just air-brushed the bad bits from my memories?

A slim figure on the skyline interrupted my thoughts. It popped up from nowhere and immediately darted down the slope towards us. By the time I had worked out that it was a runner, he had almost reached us. A moment later, he passed us, feet thudding lightly on the turf by the track, and vanished down the slope behind us. I think his singlet was red and white, but I barely had time to take it in. Meanwhile, another runner had appeared, and another; and then, after a pause, a whole line of them. They darted down towards us too quickly for comprehension, like balls of mercury, or scuttling insects disturbed by the lifting of a rock.

It was simultaneously awe-inspiring and alarming: as if we had been ambushed by a phantom army of ancient hill warriors. They streamed down at us unstoppably, skimming over the rough ground as if they were weight-less. I lost count after thirty of them, by which time our progress up the hill meant that the dozens who followed were tending to cross behind us rather than in front. But thirty was more than enough to make one obvious point with devastating force: this was proper running, utterly unlike the middle-aged pussyfooting we had been doing. These were young, vigorous runners, wearing vests and shorts: proper athletes. They had upright backs and pumping arms and made huge strides, the legs visibly pushing forward on the descents, not holding back. You could sense the eagerness in their bouncing gait, and although some would no doubt be hanging on grimly before the race was done, at this stage no one seemed to care about anything but speed.

It was hard not to feel exhilarated by the spectacle. This was fell-running as poetry, while ours was mere grown-up prose. But it was harder still to suppress another, more poignant thought: *we used to be like that*. We were runners too, once: real runners. We used to skim over mountain-sides, counting off the peaks with barely a second glance. Races like this one (I think this was the Ennerdale Horse-shoe) were how we kept ourselves sharp and tough. Charles would have been among the front-runners, and I wouldn't have been far behind. And now – well, we might as well have been looking at ghosts of our former selves.

The ghosts passed. We resumed our heavy-footed progress. Somehow we felt wearier than before. The sun-shine grew dazzling and hot, and our chatter stilled to almost nothing. We needed our energy and our breath for the remaining peaks (Brandreth, Grey Knotts, Dale Head), and all we really cared about now was making it to our self-imposed finish. But perhaps, too, a small flame of optimism had been smothered. We were still hanging in there, but we weren't the runners we used to be.

The sombre mood passed, especially when we finally arrived back in the valley we had started from. We could take the weight off our bruised legs or, if we chose, refresh ourselves with a river swim. And, once again, we felt like some of the most fortunate people in the world. The rest of the weekend was full of warmth and joy, and we vowed to repeat the experience soon, although I don't suppose we'll get round to it for ages.

But later, back at home in the lowlands of Northamptonshire, I thought about that scree, and how it seemed to slip down under my feet faster than I could run up it. And then I thought: if we do do this again, will I still be among the lucky ones who are still running? Or was that it?

2

The scrap heap

Look at me. White skin stretched thin, scuffed and fragile as perished plastic. Weary eyes. Bones too big for my muscles; hair just a bit too sparse for my forehead. Pinched lips; tightening gums. Nose skewed from some long-forgotten collision; teeth likewise. One shoulder habitually drooped: that's my mouse arm. One foot pointed slightly inwards: I've no idea why.

There was a time when an unexpected glimpse of myself in the bathroom mirror could feel fairly cheering. At least I hadn't let myself go. Nor have I since, yet that no longer helps. Today's mirror mocks me: sorry, mate, you've been let go.

My naked torso is slim, by many standards. Mainly, though, it seems not quite fully inflated. My flesh looks slack and sapless, like dried-up marzipan, and the glow of well-being I once took for granted has faded to a dim flicker, as if my batteries needed changing. Look more closely, and you'll spot a waste ground of small blemishes – unexplained scratches, slow-healing scars, rough, discoloured patches – and wild sproutings of wiry hair, some of it white, in inappropriate places.

But you're not looking closely, are you? That's the thing. You'll have gathered my problem. I'll spell it out anyway:

I'm old. There: it feels better now I've said it. Not *old* old, but still, as one soon-to-be-ex-employer told me, 'the wrong side of fifty'. Wrong side of sixty, these days, assuming that 'over' still counts as 'wrong'. I don't really see why it should, but you get tired of fighting. People will think what they think, regardless. And what they think of me these days – and perhaps of you too – is less than a four-letter-word.

Old: it's a withering label, loaded with far more meaning and judgement than the bald fact that you were born long ago. Among much else, it suggests irrelevance, as if the part of your life that mattered had already been lived. No one thinks of an old person as a work-in-progress, with skills or powers or personal qualities to be developed over time. Your story is in the past, not the future. No one will ever hire you again on the strength of your unrealised potential; and while it is still theoretically possible that on some enchanted evening a stranger will catch your eye and fall in love with you, it isn't – let's face it – very likely.

I say 'you'. I mean 'us'. Age snares us all – except the unlucky ones, who die young. Yet it can, despite being universal, drain you of your sense of belonging. It's not as bad as being marginalised for your skin colour or sexual inclination, but it's still far from pleasant. To be old, in twenty-first-century Britain, is to be guilty of a vague but repulsive depravity: to be not just frail and stale (and, in my case, pale and male) but borderline creepy. I still cringe at the memory of the moment a year or two back when I accidentally smiled at a girl – sorry, young woman – in a supermarket checkout queue . . .

But it's not just me whose smiles are stained and twisted with age. Millions of us carry the stigma. Male, female, gammon, mutton – it barely matters any more. The world has taken what it needs from us, and with each passing year we become less appetising. You don't even need to pick a question: you know already that we're not the answer. We're buzz-kills, desk-blockers, impediments to progress, health burdens waiting to happen. Our date of birth identifies us as victims, of incapacitating physical and mental decline; and yet (with annoying irony) our victimhood marks us out as culprits, too: a drag on younger, more valuable lives.

There is, of course, no appeal against such judgements, and it is only mildly consoling to reflect that, in due course, our young accusers have exactly the same thing coming to them. This is because we also know that, for all their unfairness, the prejudices of ageism are rooted, loosely, in truth. The passage of time really does dim the brilliance of youth. Bodies decay. So, often, do minds. Many of us really have passed our 'best before' date.

Some of us carry on blithely for years without noticing, but that doesn't alter the chronological facts, and in the end something always alerts us. Typically, it's a big life-event: redundancy, grandchildren, bereavement, divorce. Or it might be a health setback, or a confidence-crushing slight. But at some point, one way or another, the news gets through. You're on the old people's table now.

All this is much worse if, like me, you're a runner. That sounds narcissistic, but what do you expect? Preposterous self-pity is what runners do. It isn't the only thing we do; and, to be fair, our sport also nurtures a far more positive range of 'self'-prefixed qualities: self-reliance, self-empowerment, self-knowledge. (Sometimes I wonder whether, if it weren't for my forty-year running habit,

11

I'd have any good qualities at all.) But if you spend much time as an even moderately enthusiastic runner, you tend to develop a particular form of heightened self-awareness. Listening to our bodies, we call it, and we do it most days. Am I sickening, we wonder, or just tired? Is this the beginnings of an injury, or just healthy soreness? Above all: how much more of this can I take? Such self-examination is vital and empowers us, often, to be brave and resilient. But it easily spills over into introspection and over-sensitivity.

When our bodies start to let us down, we notice, much sooner than most, and it distresses us, acutely, because our sense of well-being tends to be intimately related to our ability to run. Sometimes, for some of us, a minor muscle strain can feel like an existential crisis.

That's how it felt for me, anyway, when a sharp pain in my ribs threatened yet another interruption to my on-off middle-aged running habit. (Four to five weeks of rest is the usual advice for an intercostal strain.) I was not quite sixty at that point, and it was the fifth time in six years that I'd been sidelined by an injury with no discernible cause. For each of the previous four (calf, groin, shoulder, Achilles tendon) a different medical practitioner had offered me some variation of the same explanation. 'Your muscles and tendons aren't as tough as they used to be,' was how the physio who treated my torn calf put it. 'There isn't really a reason. It's just age.'

I had picked myself up, eventually, from each of those setbacks, patiently helping my body to repair itself before starting again. But this time . . . Suddenly I wasn't sure I had the courage to go through it all again. Perhaps that sounds melodramatic, but that's how it felt. I seemed to be caught in a hopeless cycle of decline. After each lay-off, I had come back weaker: a little less fit, and a little less confident, and a little more prone to injury. Why would it be different this time?

It didn't help that this string of setbacks fitted easily into a wider narrative of decay. It wasn't long, for example, since my long-term job had disappeared (not just mine: two newspapers' worth), and my search for alternative employment, in my late fifties, had proved dispiritingly difficult. This wasn't unexpected. Employers have long been notorious for their collective, evidence-free belief that being over fifty makes you slow, unreliable, expensive and, in the words of one influential workplace survey, 'too old to train or reprimand'. But I was shocked by how many of the recruiters I approached simply blanked me: no interview; not even a reply. Eventually I was advised that all that experience I was boasting about on my CV was counting against me. Promising youngsters don't have forty-year employment histories. One potential employer gave it to me straight: 'Actually, we were looking for some-one younger.' I was grateful for her (illegal) honesty. But by then the message had already sunk in.

I had been hearing it from many quarters: not just potential employers but, for example, insurance compa-nies, health professionals, financial institutions. My date of birth had become a warning sign. Around the same time, I noticed I was being stalked online by advertise-ments for hearing aids and local retirement homes. When I checked this out using Google's 'Why this ad?' facility, I was told, 'This ad is based on: The time of day or your general location . . . Your age; Google's estimate of your age and interests.'

Did Google have a point? The thought began to prey on my mind. Maybe I really was on the scrapheap. The onset around the same time of the Covid-19 pandemic fuelled my insecurities. Oddly, I was less bothered by the actual dangers of a virus that predominantly killed men over sixty than by the sense that the older part of the population had acquired an extra stigma: of extreme vulnerability. It is hard to feel proud of yourself, when you have just been vaccinated against a life-threatening pandemic and your children haven't.

I tried to shrug it off. I knew that, by most standards, I had much to be grateful for. In any case, I told myself, things could be worse. But that was precisely the problem. Before long, they would be. That's what ageing means. And it struck me that, from now on, each remaining day of my life would be diminished by decay: aching joints, receding hair, weakening bladder, fumbling for my reading glasses, asking people to repeat things, wondering if I was becoming clumsier or more forgetful. In short, being a shadow of the man I used to be. I tried to remember what it felt like to look forward restlessly to the day ahead, but there was nothing there: nothing but weary regret. I had had my turn. Now it was someone else's world. Never mind a few grey hairs, I said to myself. My dreams have turned grey.

I know what you're thinking. Ageing happens. Get over it. That's what I thought, too. So I did get over it, at times, especially when I could avail myself of my usual remedy for low spirits and go for a run. But keeping that option open was a struggle. I bounced back from that rib strain, eventually, and then again, a few months later, from a shooting pain in the side of my knee. Each time, I allowed myself time to heal, did some grudging physio, tried to find other ways of keeping fit and in due course resumed running: weaker and slower, but clinging to the hope of improvement. Sometimes I could feel a little of my lost fitness returning, and there were stretches of several weeks, sometimes even months, when nothing went wrong. That happy reunion in the Lake District, mentioned in the previous chapter, coincided with such a period. Yet the good times rarely lasted – three months was about the limit – and, meanwhile, the accumulated psychological damage was slower to heal.

I had, I realised, developed a debilitating sense of my own fragility. My morning run, which for years I had thought of as my daily treat, was becoming a source of anxiety, sometimes verging on dread. Maybe it wouldn't be prudent to run right now, I would tell myself. Maybe it was more than my body could take. In any case, wasn't it too dark? Too cold? Too late already? When I did manage to drag myself out of the door, the tiniest ache or tightness would nag at my confidence. Was I about to break down again? I brooded about my performance, too. How could I have become so slow?

Every now and then, I would pull myself together. I would banish negativity, stride out with sensible vigour and reacquaint myself with the feeling that every time I ran I was making myself a little stronger. But then, just as I was starting to believe in myself again, something else would go . . .

A well-meaning relative offered what she thought was helpful advice. 'Maybe you're just too old,' she suggested. 'Maybe you should just accept that your running days are over.'

3

Play time

It's an overcast Saturday morning in September, and the world's most famous parkrun is about to begin for the 841st time. Runners of many shapes and sizes have gathered in hundreds at the southern end of Bushy Park, Teddington. The clock is ticking down towards the 9 a.m. start, and there's the usual hint of anticipatory tension creeping into the otherwise cheerful atmosphere.

In the Diana Fountain car park, however, a minute's jog away, the mood is one of uninhibited hilarity. At least, it is if you're anywhere near the bit of cardboard on a stick on which someone has written '80 AND OVER MEET HERE.'

'Are you sure you're eighty? You don't look it,' says George Frogley, not for the first time this morning, greeting yet another grizzled new arrival from beneath his placard. A few yards beyond, octogenarians are milling and bantering like over-excited children. 'Can someone remind me what we came here for?' jokes a plaintive voice. Others are discussing the fact that the key to the men's toilet appears to have been mislaid, with awkward pre-race implications for those with 'older gentleman's problems'. Luckily, the former deer park is generously dotted with mature trees.

Frogley, who is chronologically eighty-six but looks a robust sixty, is too busy dispensing goodwill to get involved in such discussions. In any case, he insists, he is not the instigator of the gathering, which he blames instead on eighty-seven-year-old Richard Pitcairn-Knowles, a retired osteopath from Sevenoaks who is currently said to be behind a tree. 'It started a few years ago,' explains Frogley. 'Richard said, come along for a jog, and it sort of grew from there.' In 2017 they persuaded eighteen over-eighties to join them on the parkrun; and the parkrun, characteristically, embraced them. By 2018 there were thirty-eight of them, and in 2019 forty-eight: all gathering to run 5 kilometres in a big, high-spirited crowd before sharing a celebratory drink and promising to do it all again next year. Coronavirus snuffed out that momentum, but there are hopes that this year's turn-out will at least be respectable.

It's hard to count confidently, because excited octogenarians resist herding. But there seem to be at least forty. Some potter distractedly into the larger crowd as soon as they have had a hand-drawn '80+' label pinned to them. Others are still catching up with old friends, or hurrying back from behind trees, when the starter instigates a round of applause for parkrun's fourth annual gathering of the over-eighties; and then, minutes later, the 5km run begins.

The 1,275 participants begin their joyous rhythmic stampede. Children sprint to the front for a few happy seconds; then the serious time-triallers take their place. The old folk are subsumed in the happy thunder of the crowd, trailed by swirling clouds of golden dust. It is impossible to keep sight of them, even by lingering right at the back: most are pressing forwards as fast as they can, and there's little to distinguish them from the younger runners around them. So I just bumble along with everyone else, enjoying the chat and the encouragement, and reflect, as many others have done in this place, on the improbability of parkrun's origins. Who could have predicted, back in 2004, that the Bushy Park Time-Trial, as it was initially called, would take root, grow, flourish and self-replicate into the Western world's fastest-growing mass participation sporting movement? Who could have imagined such a transformative and life-enhancing institution being created by a man, Paul Sinton-Hewitt, whose life in 2004 seemed defined by mid-life failure: sacked from his job, dumped by his girlfriend, sidelined from running by a broken-down body?

The contrast between his brave, generous contribution to the world and my maundering response to sensing that I was on life's scrapheap hardly needs pointing out. None the less, I feel humbled and ashamed when I think about it now, here at parkrun's birthplace, and, not for the first time, I wonder how Sinton-Hewitt found the strength to achieve what he has achieved. He was (in case his story has passed you by) a physically puny child, abandoned by his mother, tortured and bullied at school. His subsequent struggles with depression led to at least one breakdown – and yet at his lowest adult moment he turned his back on despair and did something positive. The 5km time trial he organised for his friends became a weekly fixture and, over time, a template that caught on globally, empowering millions to find their stronger selves. Did Sinton-Hewitt achieve all that in spite of the damage the world had inflicted on him? Or was it the accumulated damage that guided him to his winningly inclusive formula?

It's hard to run for long, I find, without getting distracted by random trains of thought like this. Meanwhile, the crowd has been thundering on, working its way around a wide figure of eight, over grass, hoggin path and bare earth. As the minutes go by, the chatter quietens, and the field stretches out. Beyond us, the park is already busy: with dog walkers chucking sticks, squealing children, kick-about footballers. Everywhere you look, there is play, and the world feels a warmer place for it, just as it does when yet another pair of smiling volunteer marshals ushers us in the right direction, and runner after runner pants out a breathless 'Thank you'. Which reminds me: who would have thought this world-conquering running brand – as parkrun subsequently became – would still be distinctive primarily for its commitment to compassion and inclusiveness?

But that's how it turned out. Everyone is welcome at a parkrun event: old and young, experienced or not; the slow, the sedentary and the shy just as much as the focused chasers of records and personal bests. Sinton-Hewitt, with his quiet survivor's self-belief, insisted on it, despite pressures to shift to more obviously commercial models. It isn't a race; there is no right or wrong speed to run at; anyone who finishes is a winner. This may help explain why, in this morning's throng, a few dozen octogenarians, shuffling and limping along at anything from nine-minute-mile pace to half that speed, are barely conspicuous. Everyone is part of the same trundling pack, which itself is part of a global network of hundreds of parkrun packs, all following the same empowering

Saturday-morning template. And this phenomenon is now so well-established – with seven million people registered to take part in parkrun events, in twenty-three countries, and around 350,000 actually doing so each week (140,000 of them in the UK) – that it all seems as natural, permanent and inevitable as the avenues of old oaks, limes and horse chestnuts that line our route. We pause too rarely to marvel at such benign creations, park or parkrun, or to give thanks for them.

Today, however, the air is vibrant with gratitude, especially as the octogenarians, singly and in clusters, eventually arrive at the finish. Several are visibly struggling to keep going to the end, and a casual observer might flinch at the sight of so many dusty, heavy-footed, worn-out old people. All those stoops, hunches, limps and bandages – all that weariness and resignation – suggest a defeated army. It's the precise opposite of shiny, Instagram-ready youthful perfection. But it is also the precise opposite of defeat, because in each straining gait you can discern the vigour of the soul within, and on each of those weary faces can be seen the most triumphant of smiles. 'We're just very lucky to be healthy and running at all,' says Richard Mellish, a vigorous eighty-one-year-old from Oakley, near Basingstoke, after getting his breath back.

Grubby, sweat-stained and radiant, the octogenarians potter and mingle near the finish. Some have run astonishingly fast. Graeme Baker, from Teignbridge Trotters, was fastest of all, completing the 5km course in a fraction over 28 minutes. John Holland, from Chelmsford, and Amos Seddon, from Harwich, were about half a minute behind, with Dennis Carter and Eva Osborne, both from

Wymondham, also breaking half an hour. Eva's time is a new age-group record, as is the 31:08 recorded by eighty-five-year-old Tom Harrison, from Reading.

None of these runners seems drained by the experience. Instead, they clap energetically as the 'oldies' – as eighty-year-old Hilary Bradt describes them – continue to arrive. Yogi Allen, a snowy-haired Hash House Harrier from East Grinstead, cruises in at a patient, floating plod, urged on loudly by a much younger club mate. Subsequent finishers tend to be dragging their feet, sometimes with difficulty, but bubble none the less with high spirits. Younger runners are still swarming around them, occasionally offering words of admiration or encouragement. But as time goes by the elderly predominate. They're a varied bunch, with little obvious in common beyond their '80+' labels and general air of age-related imperfection. There are lots of bald, bronzed domes, and lots of thick, bright white manes. Some of them are tall, some short, some thin, some fat. But there is one other thing they share: those smiles of childish delight.

The two ninety-year-olds – Dermot Lynch, a Bushy Park regular, and Geoff Jackson, who has come up from Didcot – both record times in the low fifties, both grinning beatifically. But the happiest finisher may be eighty-nine-year-old Albert Yee (grandfather of Olympic silver medallist triathlete Alex Yee), who plods home proudly with his walking poles in well over an hour. This is nearly half an hour slower than his previous attempt, two years earlier. But, he explains afterwards, 'I had an operation, so I'm back to square one.' Now, however, he is at square two.

By the end, it turns out, forty-two runners over eighty

have finished the 5km run, with a combined age of getting on for 3,500 years. Their average time, by my hasty calculation, is around forty-three minutes for the women (eight of them) and about forty-and-a-half for the men. But this really isn't about time – or not that kind of time, anyway.

'It's just something we enjoy doing,' says John Holland, a kindly-looking eighty-one-year-old who had driven up from Essex with his wife. His arthritic knee had behaved itself, and he was pleased to have got round without further damage. 'I've never been much good,' he adds (although I know forty-year-olds who would be satisfied with a 5km time of 28:37). 'But I enjoy it. I just plod around.'

For Richard Pitcairn-Knowles, a tall, stooped man with a seemingly permanent expression of amused perplexity, it's a question of seizing the moment. He took up running in his forties – 'I watched the first London Marathon and thought: "I ought to be doing this"' – and by his sixties had become one of the world's best cross-country runners in his age group. Now, in his late eighties, he is finding it a bit of a struggle again, and he seems disappointed with his performance today. 'Before lockdown I was taking thirty-nine minutes or so,' he says ruefully. 'This time it was almost forty-six. I was being overtaken by people who were walking.' He has no intention of giving up, however; or not until he absolutely has to. 'Competitiveness dwindles,' he explains, 'but it can be set ablaze quite unexpectedly.' As for physical frailty: 'People always worry that the really old runners might die. But that's a problem all the time when you're my age. So you might as well run.'

Eventually, the oldies and their families are persuaded to refuel nearby with '80+' cupcakes and glasses of celebratory Prosecco. This may not be optimal as sports nutrition, but it's perfect for the moment. There are speeches and photographs, and much laughter. Runner after runner singles out the organisers for effusive thanks. 'Pitcairn-Knowles, you're a liability,' says one. 'That was a very unpleasant experience.' The wide grin on the speaker's face tells the opposite story.

Beaming, head-banded Geoff Jackson, a remarkably sprightly ninety-year-old who usually offers post-run cakes to fellow parkrunners in Didcot, declares to anyone who will listen: 'I just can't stop running.' Hilary Bradt, a girlish-looking eighty, takes a more measured view. 'I keep going,' she explains later, 'because I know that if I stop it will be the end.'

Bradt, the third-fastest female octogenarian, had come up from Devon for the weekend. 'When I was travelling, I thought, "This is crazy." But it was lovely.' She's a hiker at heart rather than an athlete, with a lifelong enthusiasm for backpacking that not only strengthened her knees for life (she believes) but also led her back in the 1970s to found an influential publishing company, Bradt Travel Guides. She is still only partially retired from it, and is also an active writer and sculptor. In recent years, however, her adventurous energies have increasingly found an outlet in running, which she mainly enjoys as part of a three-woman group who call themselves the Old Crones. Her T-shirt proudly proclaims the group's name, along with its slogan: 'We do because we can.' Her fellow crones are scattered across the UK ('We have Devon Crone, Bucks Crone and Borders Crone') but they keep in touch, as so many older runners do, by digital means. 'If it wasn't for WhatsApp, where we can so easily swap stories, we wouldn't be doing this. Also, Strava has made a huge difference.' Bradt amused herself and her Twitter followers during lockdown by plotting her runs to draw dog shapes on the Strava app – which feels like a neat illustration of Karl Groos's principle that (in the usual paraphrased translation) 'We don't stop playing because we grow old; we grow old because we stop playing.'

Parkrun, Bradt adds, has been a blessing since she discovered it in 2015. 'I don't think any of us would still be running if it wasn't for that weekly challenge, and swapping times – usually "personal worsts" – and so on.' Her fellow Crones, she tells me, do their running despite some relatively serious health problems. 'They're the inspiration. I'm just exceptionally fortunate in still having serviceable legs.' She adds that her sister (Bucks Crone) 'has very little of her abdomen left' but is still planning to run the Great North Run 'with stitches still in her belly after surgery. She claims the medics told her there were no restrictions, but I don't expect they thought of asking whether she was doing the Great North Run . . .'

The Crone formula for a satisfactory old age is simple. 'It's about finding joy in what there is rather than moaning about what there isn't. I'm stiff and slow and all the rest of it, but that's the penalty of being eighty. It's still a wonderful world, and if you find it wonderful, then the fact that you feel stiff and sore and creaking doesn't matter as much as getting out there and seeing it.'

This sounds like such obvious common sense that I have to remind myself that it really isn't every day – is it? – that you see forty octogenarians and two nonagenarians all running 5km in the same place at the same time. Yet neither, perhaps, is it as freakish as some might assume. Hundreds of today's participants won't even have noticed the oldies: they were just a few more slow runners in an event in which the slow generally outnumber the fast. And while the over-eighties offer particularly emphatic contradiction of the stereotype that running is a young person's sport, there are plenty of other parkrunners who also disprove it. In 2019, across the world, there were 62,505 people aged sixty-five or over who completed at least one parkrun. Among these were 26,012 aged seventy or over, and 7,730 aged seventy-five or more. In percentage terms, the over-sixty-fives accounted for 3 per cent of the global total of parkrun participants that year, compared with 1 per cent ten years earlier (and all this at a time of rapid growth in the absolute number of participants).

Unofficial analysis suggests that, at Bushy Park, the upward trend is similar, but the proportion of older runners may be much higher. Roderick Hoffman, a retired statistician and active parkrun enthusiast, calculates that 30 per cent of finishers at parkrun's longest-standing event are now aged fifty-five or more. He speculates that the bulk of these 'were also doing parkrun ten years ago – they have simply got ten years older.' Either way, it is clear that there is no shortage of participants of pensionable age, and it therefore seems reasonable to assume that there will be plenty more active octogenarian runners coming on stream as the years go by. Frogley dreams of one day gathering 100 of them at the same event, which doesn't seem particularly unrealistic. Already, it isn't hard to identify others who might have made it to Bushy Park but didn't: people like Alan Anderson, eighty-seven, who was running his 590th parkrun in nearby Osterley that same morning, pushing his wife in a wheelchair as he usually does; or Conrad Slater, eighty-six, who was running his 235th parkrun at his usual location in Fell Foot, Cumbria. It's getting them all to the start line that's the challenge, not the actual running.

Running in old age remains rare, but it is no longer jaw-droppingly extraordinary. And while it's true that, as Hoffman puts it, 'the concept of parkrun is agreeable to the needs of the older runner,' the trend – in so far as it's measurable – goes far beyond the parkrun movement. Globally, getting on for half of all recreational running is done by people over forty, and these, too, are getting older. There's a big drop-off in participation between forty and sixty-five, but the 'survivors' – the people who are still running beyond retirement age and into their seventies and eighties – are an increasingly visible minority. In the 2021 London Marathon, for example, 471 of the finishers of the actual and virtual events were over seventy: 145 women and 326 men. More than a hundred of these were over seventy-five, and seventeen were over eighty.

Reliable information about wider participation is patchy. Until recently, no one thought to ask about the running habits of pensioners. But Sport England's big ongoing Active Lives survey suggests that, in 2020–21, there were 198,800 English adults over sixty-five (1.9 per cent of adults in their age group) who ran at least twice a month, and 31,600 in the seventy-five-to-eighty-four age range (0.8 per cent) who did the same. This would suggest a UK-wide figure of about 236,000 relatively regular runners over sixty-five – of whom around 37,500 are aged between seventy-five and eighty-four. That's a

significant proportion in a general UK running population of about 2.5 million. The number of twice-a-month
runners aged eighty-five or over appears to be too small
and variable to provide a reliable statistic, but there are
probably hundreds and perhaps even more. In 2022,
RunBritain, the licensing body for all races authorised
by UK Athletics, had 1,736 over-eighties and 115
over-nineties recorded on its database of 572,507 active,
competitive runners who had taken part in UKA-
licensed races at any point in the twelve years since 2010.
These are cumulative totals, of course, but the only
runners who show up in RunBritain's figures are the
keen minority who actually race. So perhaps if you threw
in every last jogger, the levels of eighty-plus participation in any given year wouldn't be so different from the
figures I've quoted.

Back-of-an-envelope extrapolations from these and
other sources suggest that runners keen enough to run
once a week or more are much rarer: perhaps barely
50,000 of those 236,000 twice-a-monthers over sixty-
five; and, by extension, about 7,500 over-seventy-fives.
Fewer still compete in races. Yet it appears that, even so,
before Covid, there may have been as many as 380,000
race-entering runners worldwide who were sixty-five or
over, with many times more (presumably) running regularly without competing.

Even these figures are tiny, relative to the wider population. But the messages are big and unambiguous. Lots
of people run when they're in their forties: roughly one
in seven. It simply isn't unusual. But only a few – perhaps
one in fifty – will still be running when they're sixty-five;
and even fewer will keep going into serious old age. There

are 12.7 million Britons aged sixty-five or over, and 98.1 per cent of them are not runners.

There are of course two ways of reading these numbers. They tell us that most people can't keep running in much later life. They also prove that some people can. The odds are against us, but it can be done. And the message from Bushy Park's annual gathering of octogenarians is that, for those who do keep going, the rewards appear to be just as rich in terms of joy, companionship, well-being and laughter as they were at earlier stages of life. As improbable but just-about-achievable sporting targets go, this is not a bad one to aim at.

It's also worth remembering that the elderly runners in those statistics were born long ago. My generation – the running boomers now within sight of retirement – have much more reason to think of 'whole life running' as a realistic possibility. We are less likely than our parents' generation to die young; more likely to be keen runners in the first place; and a lot less likely to be deterred from running in later life for fear of ridicule. This is especially true of women, whose rarity in the oldest cohorts (210 registered UK female runners over eighty, nine over ninety) echoes their lack of sporting opportunities when they were younger. Future cohorts will have higher expectations, and fewer inhibitions.

Meanwhile, already, late-life running and mid-life running are on the increase, which is more than can be said of early-life running. Maybe the London 2012 Olympics really did succeed in its declared aim to 'inspire a generation': it just wasn't the generation the organisers had in mind. The difference, I suppose, is that we oldies and oldies-in-waiting have often experienced the life-enhancing benefits of a running habit already. Of course we want to keep going for the rest of our lives. Why wouldn't we?

The odds may be against us, in any individual case, but it's a statistical certainty that some British runners of my vintage will prove as durable as the Bushy Park octogenarians, when our turn comes. Some of us will grow up to be as active, energetic and inspiring as Pitcairn-Knowles, Frogley, Yee, Bradt and the rest. Why shouldn't I be among them?

This seems like a worthwhile aspiration. But the long-term goal is only part of the attraction. As with many running goals, the real reward comes from the excitement, motivation and energy you can derive simply from setting your sights on it and travelling hopefully towards it. I am still nearly two decades short of the octogenarian stage of my life, and have many more immediate aspirations (including staying alive through my sixties and seventies). But the thought of celebrating my eightieth birthday with a run or a race – and spending the intervening years being fit enough to make that feasible – fills me with an enthusiasm for the long-term future that I haven't felt in a long while. Maybe that enthusiasm could brighten my more immediate future as well.

Statistically, it remains unlikely that I – or you – will make it through the physiological minefield of our sixties and seventies without losing the ability to run. But we can enjoy trying. And we may even find that, with the right expert guidance, we can adjust the odds in our favour.

4

The parting of ways

In a cluttered fourth-floor office near London Bridge, in one of the massive red-brick buildings of Guy's Campus, at King's College's Centre for Human & Applied Physiological Sciences, a middle-aged professor called Stephen Harridge takes a break from a fraught afternoon of funding applications for his Ageing Research at King's (ARK) programme to talk me through the basics of the physiology of ageing.

'Look at these curves,' he says, opening his laptop and calling up a series of his favourite graphs. These plot the decline of world track records set by older athletes, through successive five-year age groups from 35–39 to 75–79, in disciplines from 100 metres to 10,000 metres. It seems like rather a narrow focus, but this, says Harridge, is what makes the data important. At ARK, he explains, 'we study the actual process of ageing. If you just study a random group of old people, it's impossible to know what's caused by ageing and what's down to other things. There are so many contaminants, relating to poor diet, alcohol use, smoking, and above all physical inactivity.' Such factors are ubiquitous in developed societies, but they are not normal. 'The body was designed to be active.

If you're interested in the biological process of human ageing, you have to study physically active people.'

Harridge himself is a former junior international athlete, a 400m hurdler of the same hurdling vintage as Colin Jackson and Sally Gunnell. ('But I wasn't nearly as good.') His main long-term colleague, Emeritus Professor Norman Lazarus, is an athlete too: an eighty-four-year-old competitive cyclist who is involved in ARK's research as both scientist and guinea pig. But ARK's focus on Masters athletes – a term that typically embraces anyone over thirty-five, all the way up to extreme old age, who actively trains to compete in athletic competitions at any level – isn't really about athletics. It's about ageing.

With these record graphs, explains Harridge, what you see is the trajectory of unavoidable ageing. Whatever the discipline, the curve slopes downward with age in much the same way: gently at first, with a dramatically steepening decline near the very end. 'These are people who are in the best physical condition it's possible to be in – and this is the decline that you get resulting purely from age.'

Such data is valuable not just because of the relative lack of 'contaminants' but because, being based on competitive performance, it shows change in all-round physiological performance rather than a specific function such as muscle power or respiration. If you're going to set a world record, 'everything needs to be functioning perfectly. You've got to have good cognitive processing, good cardiovascular and respiratory function, good balance, good neuromuscular function. It all has to be integrated and working well.' Yet even when you isolate individual elements, they tend to decline (with minor variations) along much the same trajectory.

What makes the curve dramatic is the contrast that appears when you put it on a graph where two other groups of people are also represented: regular, non-elite exercisers; and the sedentary. The non-elite exercisers are in a broad 'green zone'. Their functionality is at a much lower absolute level than the elite, but it declines with age along a more-or-less parallel curve, sloping gently before sinking sharply down to zero (representing death) at the end. In both cases, these ageing exercisers spend most of their old age above the horizontal line representing 'loss of independence'. The 'gold zone' elite are much further above this independence line – and can of course run faster, throw further, jump higher and generally do more exciting and impressive things than the normal exercisers. But they differ only slightly from the green zone group in the length of the very short period, just before death, when their physiological functionality sinks below the independence line. Both groups experience the same 'compressed morbidity'.

The really striking difference appears in the big red area below the green zone, with a series of irregular white zigzags across it representing the uncertain health trajectories that result from 'non-inherent ageing'. This is what awaits the sedentary majority, for whom ageing interacts with the effects of inactivity to let in a sea of physiological troubles, resulting in many long years, sometimes decades, below the independence threshold. It's impossible to predict the detail, but the broad effect is clear: 'extended morbidity' – a large, grey, twilight zone, sometimes decades long, in which life starts to blur into death.

None of this is controversial. It's what you'd expect: a causal link between regular physical activity and high levels of functionality in old age. Yet to see it set out so starkly is to wonder why on earth anyone in a position to choose would opt to be in the red zone.

The obvious answer is that we don't. No one would make such a choice – not consciously. Yet neither is it necessarily beyond our control.

On the other side of the world, in Vancouver, Canada, Dr Angela Brooks-Wilson, head of the Healthy Ageing Study at Canada's Michael Smith Genome Sciences Centre (part of the BC Cancer Research Centre), has spent much of the past twenty-five years trying to unlock the secrets of healthy ageing. Her specific professional interest is in the genetics of cancer susceptibility, but she has also overseen some of the world's most comprehensive research into what she calls 'Super Seniors' – that is, people over eighty-five who have never been diagnosed with cancer, cardiovascular disease, major pulmonary disease, diabetes or dementia. Her as-yet-uncompleted mission is to identify what it is that such people have in common.

It's a question with an obvious answer: this tiny minority – roughly 2 per cent of their cohort – are people who have drawn winning tickets in the lottery of later life. Their health is robust, they have avoided catastrophic accidents, and, as a result, they are relatively undamaged by age – and well-placed to survive and thrive into their nineties and beyond. But what lies behind this good fortune? The various studies that Brooks-Wilson has overseen, starting with the first big Super Seniors study from 2004–7, suggest that these 'super' individuals possess certain common traits. They show above-average levels of cognitive and physical functionality, and below-average levels of depression. They tend to have had relatively long-lived parents. They are less likely than non-'super' seniors to be neurotic and more likely to be physically active. And they are more likely to be extroverted, open, agreeable, conscientious and, as Brooks-Wilson puts it, to be 'very engaged in life, doing lots of things'.

These observations hint at the possibility that by modifying our behaviour we might improve our chances of becoming Super Seniors ourselves (although we can't do much about our parents). But it is only a possibility. We don't really know what the information means. Are these traits and habits a cause of the Super Seniors' physiological good fortune? Or are they merely an effect?

There's a similar ambiguity at a cellular level. Most Super Seniors are notable for having telomeres – the protein caps that seal the ends of our chromosomes – that are a very specific length, slightly (but not dramatically) longer than average. This is a clear biological marker: they are physiologically different from most of us. But, again, what does this mean? Telomere lengths are set at birth and in most species correlate directly to lifespan: if your telomeres are short, your life is unlikely to be long. But they can also be affected by life events and, as a result, are symptoms as much as determinants of how well you will age. A study at the Universidade Católica de Brasília, led by Samuel da Silva Aguiar and published in the *International Journal of Sports Medicine* in 2021, showed that Masters athletes had longer telomere lengths (and healthier levels of insulin and the SIRT1 protein) than non-athletes. But was this the result of their active habits – or the cause, the thing about them that predisposed them to be active in later life?

Another Canadian, Mark Tarnopolsky, a sixty-year-old professor of Pediatrics and Medicine at McMaster University in Hamilton, Ontario (who also happens to be a top-class adventure racer, winter triathlete and ski orienteer), argues that the evidence is overwhelming. 'There's no question,' he says. 'It's not like, oh, you're just lucky, because you had long telomeres. Telomeres are longer in those that are well-trained athletes. We all have the same length telomeres when we start, but training stimulates the production of an enzyme called telomerase, and that helps maintain telomere length.'

But Brooks-Wilson is convinced that, in addition, some kind of hereditary key to late-life well-being will be identified one day: a genetic idiosyncrasy that explains why a charmed minority are more likely to be age-resistant than the rest of us. It won't be an obvious one, because it turns out that – with a few specific exceptions (for example, the APOe4 variant associated with Alzheimer's) – Super Seniors are no less likely than ordinary people to have the common undesirable genetic variants associated with the big, bad diseases that they have none the less avoided. But it may be a protective one: a genetic buffer or buffers to negate the effects of the dangerous variants.

'That would be the holy grail,' she smiles. 'An age-resistant gene: something that really protects against ageing. And if we found that, we would want to mimic that with a drug . . .'

You can see why this might be an attractive prospect – and not just for the humanitarian reasons that motivate Brooks-Wilson. Globally, we spend £250 billion a year on anti-ageing products. Imagine what we'd spend on a product that worked.

Yet even Brooks-Wilson, whose life's work is founded on the proposition that there is a genetic defence against ageing waiting to be discovered, concedes that the most important buffers that have protected the Super Seniors in her studies from serious disease may not be genetic at all. It might simply come down to the way they have chosen to live. 'Genetics,' says Brooks-Wilson, 'is the small part of the story. Healthy ageing is probably of the order of about twenty-five per cent genetic. The rest of the story is lifestyle.'

Anything in particular? 'Well, the big one that we know about is quitting smoking. A lot of the Super Seniors used to smoke, because that's what people did back then, but it was only the quitters who survived.' And after that? 'Exercise, probably.'

Put like that, it sounds like a hunch, but it's a well-established fact. Exercise slows down the physiological deterioration associated with ageing. It isn't always easy to quantify its effects precisely, because other big lifestyle choices (on diet, smoking, alcohol, etc.) play a part as well; and exercise, of course, takes many forms. But in so far as the picture can be clarified – in Steve Harridge's graphs, for example – the difference it makes is striking. Some studies have even suggested that a sedentary lifestyle is worse for your health than smoking.

This shouldn't surprise us. 'We are essentially hunter-gatherers in a modern society,' says Janet M. Lord, Professor of Immune Cell Biology at the University of Birmingham. 'Food is readily available, and we are sedentary most of the time, and that is not how we have evolved. We have evolved to be physically very active and not to eat meals all the time.'

Like Harridge, Lord, who is sixty-three, used to be a serious athlete, although her competitive career was ended by a broken pelvis in her early forties. 'I still run, but I'm not doing the distance any more – well, just a few marathons – and I've really slowed down recently.' She is in no doubt, however, about the benefits of keeping the habit going. 'Much of what we consider normal ageing is actually due to inactivity.'

In 2018 Lord collaborated with Harridge, Lazarus and others on a study that illustrated this dramatically. The project focused on 125 keen cyclists, male and female, aged fifty-five to seventy-nine, none of them Olympians but all of them serious enough to be able to cycle 100km in less than six-and-a-half hours, if they were men, or 60km in less than five-and-a-half hours if they were women. 'We thought, well, we'll basically look at everything. You name it, they spent three days in the lab with us, and we researched it. And lots of things that any medical textbook would say, this is what happens in old age, just doesn't happen in these guys.'

They weren't entirely age-proof. 'Lung function (VO$_2$ max) had still declined, and the maximum heart rate they could achieve still declined. But the values were still very high' – in some cases equivalent to inactive adults thirty-five years younger. In other respects, meanwhile, they didn't seem to have declined at all. 'Things like immunity didn't decline. They didn't get an increase in blood pressure, their insulin resistance didn't decline, and there was no increase in cholesterol, no change in blood lipids.'

The findings relating to the immune system, Lord's speciality, were particularly striking. Usually the thymus, which regulates the immune system and produces new T-cells, becomes significantly less effective from your early fifties onwards. 'So your immune system deteriorates. You get a build-up of senescent T-cells: old T-cells that can increase inflammation. They are just not very good at their job, basically. Meanwhile the thymus, which produces T-cells in the first place, atrophies with age. So the generation of new T-cells declines, and the proportion of senescent T-cells increases steadily.'

In many old people, this results in a phenomenon known as 'inflammaging': a state of chronic inflammation that can explode into deadly cytokine storms; it has also been linked to the terrible death-toll of Covid-19 among older age groups.

In the keen Masters cyclists, however, this failure of immune system functionality didn't happen. Instead, 'they were producing just as many T-cells as the healthy but inactive twenty-to-thirty-six-year-olds in the control group.'

Subsequent reports suggested that the oldest cyclists, including Norman Lazarus, had 'the immune systems of twenty-year-olds'. This wasn't quite true. 'Some aspects of immunity do decline,' says Lord. 'You still get a build-up of senescent T-cells that are not very good at their job. But the Masters cyclists had a good thymus, so they had lots of new T-cells as well, so they're less prone to out-of-control inflammation.' Part of their secret, it seems, was that they had managed by sheer hard work to minimise age-related loss of muscle mass – because muscle, when exercising, produces myokines that help regulate the immune system.

The news reports also extrapolated from the study the idea that, as one headline put it, 'exercise can reverse ageing.' But this wasn't exactly true either. The study showed that, to a large extent, exercise can reverse the effects of physical inactivity; ageing, by definition, is the decline that remains. But the extent of the reversal is, none the less, dramatic, and so is the implication that it is available to any of us.

'We're not saying: "Look at these amazing old people with their incredible VO$_2$ max,"' said Harridge, when I talked to him about the same study back in London, 'because actually these old people are where they should be. Physical activity isn't an intervention. Inactivity is the intervention.'

Just to be clear, you don't need to be physically active in order to live for a long time. That's fairly likely to happen anyway. The demographic trends are overwhelming. I was born (in 1960) with a life-expectancy of just over sixty-eight years. A British child born today would have a projected lifespan roughly two decades longer: 87.6 for a boy and 90.2 for a girl. Even I, having survived to reach my early sixties, can now expect to continue to eighty-five; and if you live in the UK and have just reached your sixty-fifth birthday, you should consider yourself unlucky if you don't now get within sight of ninety.

Such extensions have been replicated all over the world (often from a lower base), and the biggest pandemic of the modern age has so far caused barely a ripple in the rising demographic tide. In 1960, global average lifespan was around fifty-three years; by 2022, it was getting on for seventy-three. Climate change, pandemics and war may yet reverse the trend, but in the developed world it feels like a long-term adjustment. By 2030, one person in six will be over sixty. Life beyond retirement is no longer a footnote. It is a whole chapter; perhaps even a whole new volume. Worldwide, there are 617 million people aged sixty-five or over; by 2050, there are expected to be 1.6 billion, including roughly a third of the population of Europe and, I hope, me. (All I have to do in order to still be around then is reach my ninetieth birthday, or thereabouts: something which, according to the Office for National Statistics, I now have a better than one-in-four chance of doing.)

But that's only half the story. Longevity, the baby-boom generation's most startling blessing, is also its quiet curse. That final chapter or volume of life that begins around the time we retire from the workplace will, for all too many of us, be a bleak one. This is because health-span – that part of your life before bodily deterioration starts limiting your ability to live independently – has failed to keep pace with our extended lifespans. Of the 12 million people in the UK aged sixty-five and over, more than six million suffer from two or more chronic illnesses. Around 3.5 million are unable to perform at least one of the basic 'activities of daily living', such as eating, dressing, bathing or going to the toilet; getting on for two million suffer from moderate or severe frailty and, as a result, reduced mobility. Not all these millions are the same millions, of course, but they tend to overlap, and the older you get, the more likely they are to overlap in you. It's the same with other age-related afflictions. Roughly three million old people in the UK suffer from depression; around six million rely mainly on television or pets for company. And that's before you consider the various forms of dementia, which currently afflict one person in fourteen (about 860,000) over the age of sixty-five – and one in six over eighty.

That's what the future holds for us collectively: hundreds of millions of life-years made miserable by age-related ill-health. The average woman is unwell for nineteen years at the end of her life, the average man for sixteen. But it doesn't happen to everybody. A fortunate minority will remain mobile, independent and free from chronic pain until almost the end.

Which group will you end up in? It's a big question. When Benjamin Disraeli claimed in 1845 that Britain had become 'two nations', he had in mind the gulf between the rich and the poor, 'who are as ignorant of each other's habits, thoughts, and feelings, as if they were . . . inhabitants of different planets'. A comparable gulf is opening up today between two different subspecies of old people: the fortunate and the unfortunate. Both experience an unprecedentedly long stretch of life beyond traditional retirement age – getting on for a quarter of their time on earth. For one group, this extended twilight darkens rapidly into a chronic struggle with illness, pain, isolation and immobility; for the fortunate remainder, life remains healthy, active and full of barely diminished possibility until almost the very end.

As with many life-shaping questions of collective identity (gender, race, nationality, class), which group you end up in is largely a matter of luck. Your future selects you, not the other way round. Yet it's not just that. Where old age is concerned you can, to a surprising extent, make your own luck.

*

'If physical activity were a drug,' said the UK's then Chief Medical Officer, Dame Sally Davies, in 2017, 'we would refer to it as a miracle cure.' It isn't, so we don't; but the miracle remains. As the Stanford physician and octogenarian runner Walter Bortz II put it several decades earlier: 'There is no drug in current or prospective use that holds as much promise for sustained health as a lifetime programme of physical exercise.'

It's that simple: old people who keep fit have the physical and mental attributes of much younger people; or rather, if Harridge and Lord are to be believed, old people who don't keep fit have the physical and mental attributes of even older people. Throw in a few other common-sense lifestyle choices, and you have a formula of spectacular effectiveness. Long-term runners can expect to live seven years longer than average, and a fifty-year-old who doesn't smoke, drinks alcohol only moderately, has a balanced diet, maintains a healthy weight and exercises for at least half an hour a day can expect, on average, around a decade of extra health-span compared with a fifty-year-old who ticks none of those boxes. A physically and mentally active lifestyle also delays the onset of the most common form of dementia (fronto-temporal dementia): for the most active quarter of the population, its onset is 55 per cent slower.

The formula is fallible. Disease, accidents and other misfortunes strike down the tirelessly athletic as well as the sedentary and self-destructive, and around 25 per cent of healthy ageing is, as we know, genetic. It is all too easy to become miserably inactive in later life for reasons entirely beyond your control. When you're still at the planning stage, however, it's a no-brainer. Of course you should aspire to be in the green zone rather than the red zone.

What I still found puzzling, however, was what we stand to gain from being in the gold zone rather than the green zone. Why go to all the effort of becoming a top Masters athlete, if you can enjoy the same benefits by being an ordinary regular exerciser?

Harridge drew my attention back to his first graph. 'We're all declining. We're all going to die. What matters is how well you can function in the meantime. In the gold zone, you're still going to lose functionality at much the same rate as someone in the green zone. But look at where you're declining from.' Just as skydivers say that 'altitude is safety' (because the higher you are when something goes wrong, the more scope you have for taking action to prevent the catastrophe that otherwise awaits you at ground level), so, for the old, fitness is youth. The higher your level of physical functionality, the further you can fall without crashing through the 'loss of independence' line.

Gold zone athletes also tend to enjoy breadth of functionality – that is, most things work. They can find their way to competitions, get to the start line at the right time, hear the starting gun, run without over-balancing, and so on. This provides an extra level of health security. 'The trouble with having a smaller number of things working well is that you only need one part of the system to sink below a certain level and you get problems of functionality that derail the entire system.'

In terms of simple cardiovascular risk, hard-core athletic training appears to offer little or no advantage over a generally active lifestyle (an observation confirmed by the publication in 2021 of a major five-year randomised study of septuagenarians in Trondheim, Norway). But that broader, all-round functionality gives the athletes an advantage. If you lack the upper body strength to get out of your chair, says Harridge, it doesn't matter how good your heart, lungs and legs are. 'If you can't get up, you can't do it.'

No one can resist the onslaught of ageing for ever, but athletes in the gold zone tend to be last to succumb: partly because of the breadth and depth of their training, but also because of the extra motivation that competitive sport provides. The trouble with the kind of moderate exertion that keeps you in the green zone is that, after a while, the thrill wears off. The sense of well-being you are used to associating with exercise gives way to aches and pains; the buzz of competition gives way to sensible keep-fit routines. Of course you lose interest – and it's no surprise to learn that, in the 65–74 age group, only one Briton in ten does the recommended amount of aerobic and muscle-strengthening exercise. Nothing matters more than your health once you've lost it, but until that point it's a rather abstract concern, and thoughts about long-term benefits are easily obscured by the more press-ing concerns of the present. Even Harridge, for all his passion and understanding, finds it hard to practise what he preaches. 'I do try,' he said, 'but it's hard to find the time. I have a long commute . . .'

But sporting competition, which can go well or badly depending on how conscientiously you train: that could be a different matter. Harridge's eyes lit up when I sug-gested that perhaps he himself could return to competitive hurdling, after a twenty-year break. 'I'd have to be very careful,' he mused. 'There'd be a lot of ground to make up.

But, then again, I've probably benefited from not having the wear and tear. Maybe I should . . .'

That's the thing, I thought. Maybe he should. Maybe I should too. Something must be happening in the gold zone; and if nothing else, perhaps its inhabitants could teach me something.

5

Neverland

Early one bright September morning, I crawled out of a tent in an unfamiliar corner of northern Italy, hoping that the crunching of my joints wouldn't wake my fellow campers. I padded my way to the beach and began, very gently, to run.

The pale sun was barely higher than the beach-side pines, but the quiet sea was already glittering. Inland, hazy, snow-capped peaks floated on a blue horizon. I jogged sleepily towards them, muscles still cold from the night, barefoot on the sand, until the mouth of a canal blocked my way. A fisherman, still as wood, sat at the water's edge. I noticed him only as I turned away.

Retracing my steps, I raised my pace and my gaze – and gasped at what now lay ahead: a mile or more of sandy beach, straight and empty, with the Adriatic shining on one side and, on the other, the once-fashionable resort town of Caorle, sleeping behind a canvas-and-plastic battalion of vacant sunloungers. For a worn-out runner like me, this was paradise: no stress, no pressure; just a chance to enjoy being out in the fresh morning, moving as nature intended. I planted my feet as neatly as I could – these were the day's first footprints – and immersed myself in the moment: damp sand underfoot, the sun gently warming my back, the lazy sighs of the waves.

I hadn't run so happily for months, and the further I ran, the more I felt myself glowing with a mixture of well-being and self-satisfaction. How could I ever have considered myself washed up? This was real running: natural running. And, I told myself, I was doing it rather well, especially for a man of my age.

Then I spotted a moving figure on the promontory ahead. It skipped down rapidly from the sea wall to the sand, revealing itself as a runner. It was a man, solitary and noiseless as me. He sped towards me, following, like me, the wet margin between beach and sea. Soon we could see one another's faces. Our paths crossed. We exchanged the customary grunts and nods. Then he was gone – yet his image stayed in my mind.

Like me, he was barefoot and shirtless. Unlike me, he was old. No, hang on: I'm old too. Perhaps he had noticed my age, as I had his. But he seemed older – or older than my imagined self. His cropped hair was entirely white; his face lined and leathery. His tanned body was fit: fatless (unlike mine) and writhing with muscles. On reflection, the vigour of his running suggested that he was younger than me. Yet you couldn't have mistaken him for a young man. His body had the same faded quality I had previously noted in myself: a thinness to the skin, a sparseness to the chest hair, a hint of skeleton in the collarbone and shoulders. I hate to think what impression I made on him.

I was still pondering this, wondering if he was in his fifties, sixties or seventies, when I noticed another figure approaching, female and seemingly sprinting. At least, she was pumping her knees and elbows, staring eyes focused on the space in front. I don't think she even noticed my nod and grunt. This was proper, performance-maximising training, unlike my sleepy tourist's jog. Again, however, she was hard to place on the age spectrum. Wisps of white hair protruded from her bright headscarf, and her face was stretched like a pensioner's; yet her animated gaze and gait suggested a surfeit of youthful energy.

At the promontory I climbed up to the cobbled sea wall, and was distracted as I ran along it by a view of the round, brown-brick cathedral bell tower, which still rises from the town's untidy sea of red-tiled roofs, exactly as it has for nine centuries. It was hard to look at it without feeling drawn into the distant past, and by the time my thoughts returned to the present, I was already descending to the next stretch of beach, where two other runners were picking their way up towards me: a wizened, open-shirted man whose tentative jogging could have been that of an eighty-year-old, give or take a decade; and another white-haired woman, in a blue 'Italia' T-shirt, whose bouncing gait seemed implausible for anyone much over forty.

So it continued: more runners on the beach beyond; more still when I retraced my steps; and more uncertainty about where each one fitted into the age spectrum. One or two may have been younger than me, but many would in any other context have been described as 'elderly'. Sometimes the wrinkles said mid-seventies while the powering legs said mid-forties. All I could conclude with confidence was that they were proper athletes; and that, whatever else they were, they weren't young.

By the time I glimpsed the trees by my campsite again,

the coast was swarming with such runners. They weren't doing anything organised: just taking advantage of the flat space, each in their own way. But the collective impression they made was startling: like hyper-active crabs scuttling on the drying sand. Sunlight glinted from silver hair and golden-bald scalps, and it occurred to me that, in the UK, most of these people would be entitled to free public transport.

It was as if I had stumbled into a lost land, whose old people are mysteriously untouched by age. And one unwelcome effect of this was that I kept being overtaken, often with withering ease. Usually I strive desperately to avoid being passed, but this felt like a morning for pretending not to notice or care. I did put in a final spurt just before the campsite, but even that didn't prevent a woman who reminded me of my mother from casually speeding past me.

It was a relief to stop and catch my breath. I felt chastened, for obvious reasons; but mainly I felt reassured. I was in the right place.

As the day progressed, and I took up my duties at the stadium, there would be many more old runners; and more still over the next two weeks. Altogether, more than 8,300 older athletes were in town, from forty-three European nations, supported by many further thousands of family, friends, coaches, managers and medics – and a handful of volunteers like me. Actually, they were spread between three towns: Caorle and the neighbouring settlements of Jesolo and Eraclea. But there were more than enough visitors to go round.

None of the athletes, and few of the supporters, were

younger than thirty-five. Most were pensioners, or at least of pensionable age; hundreds were in their eighties or nineties. If it wasn't quite the care home demographic, it was certainly the kind of age spectrum you'd expect to find on an ocean cruise. But no one here was sitting quietly or snoozing in a deckchair.

This, declared the banners on Caorle's stadium, was the European Masters Athletics Championships – an event of bewildering complexity, with twenty-seven different age/gender categories and up to fifty-five different events per category, distributed between the three towns apparently at random. The volunteers had been recruited to ease the competitors' visitor experience, but in Caorle, at least, we were mostly occupied with last-minute construction work and in any case were clueless, since our promised induction had failed to materialise. No one seemed surprised. This was a festival of enthusiasm rather than efficiency. And if many of the banners appeared to me to have been hung the wrong way round, so that the passing public couldn't see them, that just showed how naïve I was. This wasn't being staged for the public's benefit.

When the sporting action began, my responsibilities broadened to include such duties as hurdle moving, sandpit raking and retrieving hammers and javelins. These meant that I missed any number of events that the initiated would have considered important. But they did provide some excellent vantage points for my first close-up views of proper, organised, competitive old people's sport.

I barely knew what to make of it. Half the athletes were younger than me; some were getting on for twenty-five years younger. It seemed ridiculous to look to them for lessons about late life's challenges. Even so, their efforts impressed me. In the women's 100m, for example, Germany's Sinah Flo Haenssler-Hug won the 35–39 age group in 12.58 seconds. (The men's equivalent, held in the Jesolo stadium, was won by Team GB's Jonathan Browne in 10.94 seconds.) That's pretty fast, when you're well past a sprinter's peak. Yet somehow, from where I was standing, the events in these age groups felt tame: like a slowed-down Olympics, without the razzmatazz or significance. The competitors warmed up ferociously, just as 'real' athletes do, and psyched themselves up with shouts and grunts. They neurotically checked run-ups, equipment and judges' decisions. And they ran with great grace, speed and passion. But nobody else seemed to care. The small stadium was barely quarter-full.

As the events crept up through the age categories, however, a sense of drama crept in, and when the athletes were significantly older than me, I found myself watching with increasingly visceral engagement. This was perverse, because the performances were worse. 'Slower, lower, weaker' would be an appropriate motto. Yet I clearly wasn't alone in my perversity. The older the competitors, the more people watched.

As the days passed, familiarity tempered my fascination; but there was much to get used to. At first, I would watch anxiously if I saw an athlete in their seventies or eighties struggling to take off their tracksuit or wincing as they tied their shoes. It was like watching a care-home resident fumbling with a cardigan. Should I intervene, I wondered? But in due course I realised that such sights are commonplace in Masters athletics. Old joints creak, and range of motion declines even in the very fit. But anyone who considers themselves mobile enough to have a go on the track is, by definition, mobile enough.

One evening, I witnessed eight women's 400m finals in quick succession, starting with the W40s and working up to W80. It was like watching an animated version of that endlessly reproduced 'March of Progress' illustration in which Rudolph Franz Zallinger attempted to show how an early ape evolved in stages into modern Homo Sapiens. In this case, however, it was the March of Age. In the younger categories – won by Germany's Maren Schott in 58.64 seconds for W40 and by Sweden's Jenny Akervall in 1:01.64 in the W45 – the age factor was barely noticeable. The athletes punched the ground with their feet, sprang forward with bounce and aggression, and sprinted in the final stages as if they were floating above the track. If it hadn't been for the underwhelming applause from the half-empty stands, you could have mistaken it for an elite international meeting at the ordinary senior level.

By the time it got to W50 (won by Spain's Esther Colas in 1:02.16), you could see how the years were taking their toll. Many runners seemed to be plugging on bravely rather than sprinting without restraint, and the gaps between the competitors were growing. Great Britain's Virginia Mitchell won the W55 convincingly (in 1:04.73) with a vigorous and fluid run that looked as though it belonged in a younger age group, but her rivals seemed to be treating it as a contest of stamina rather than speed. Mitchell, who had discovered Masters twenty years earlier, soon after having her first baby, would also win the 800m four days later. She later told me that she was running with a chronic heel injury – an insertional Achilles problem – but 'I decided not to think about it.' Back in England, it would take her nearly a year to recover.

Meanwhile, as the long Caorle afternoon faded into evening, the one-lap finals continued. In the W60 (won by Norway's Annie Undheim in 1:10.46) the strides were shorter and stiffer. I don't suppose anyone was consciously trying to spare their joints the pain of maximum impact, but that's how it looked. There was less knee lift, less heel lift, less elasticity; jerkier movements; more visible struggle. It was still a lot more athletic than it would have been had I been doing the running. Yet, seen so soon after the younger age groups, it put me in mind of a parents' race at school.

Great Britain's Caroline Powell looked recognisably like an elite quarter-miler – albeit an unhurried one – when winning the W65 in a European record of 1:08.67, but it was hard to say the same of some of those she beat. The nearest was nearly 3 seconds behind. By the W70, won by France's Michelle Peroni in 1:19.18, it was hard to imagine that you were watching anything but old people; although, to be fair, even an 80-second 400m is hardly jogging. The raw muscular power that pulsated from the earlier races was absent; instead, that apparent reluctance to hammer stiff joints too violently had become more pronounced, and perhaps in the posture of one or two runners there was the hint of a stoop. Strangely, however, it wasn't dull – especially if you watched the runners' faces. These were, after all, what would conventionally be called old ladies, yet they were running with the vigour of forty-year-olds and the competitive hunger of twenty-year-olds. In the home straight, you could see them pressing themselves fiercely against the limits of self-inflicted pain, and their courage was all the more magnificent because of their relative frailty.

The W75 and W80 finals raced together, since they had only five finalists between them. Rietje Dijkman, a cheerful, bespectacled churchgoer from Amsterdam, won the W80 with a world record of 1:29.84, well ahead of the Swedish W75 winner, Kristina Carlsson, whose time was 1:39.57. The fact that one or two runners seemed to doubt their ability to complete the distance at all added depth to the drama. At one point, as the line of runners began to stretch out, I found myself imagining the group as a vast, slow-moving insect, angular and relentless. Then they strung out further still, on the far side of the track, and the muscular Dijkman – her strawberry-blonde hair almost matching her orange Netherlands vest – pulled away into what would eventually be a 50-metre lead. And I realised that the remaining runners now reminded me of something stranger: the final 'dance of Death' scene of Ingmar Bergman's cinematic masterpiece, *The Seventh Seal*. That's the one in which Death, hooded and sickle-bearing, can be seen leading a line of silhouetted figures along a windswept horizon – and everything else we have learnt about the characters fades against the irresistible reality of their mortality. In print, the comparison seems ludicrous. Perhaps it was. But the shadows were lengthening, and the light was fading, and to me at that moment the race seemed to have as much to do with the human condition – ageing, vulnerability, dying – as with a mere scramble for medals.

It hardly needs saying that, for the athletes themselves, such fanciful responses can be deeply irritating. It *is* about medals, they'll tell you, and about times and finishing positions; and it's frustrating that the public doesn't pay more attention to their considerable achievements in these respects. But the public has grasped something else: that the most dramatic struggle of Masters athletics is with age itself. If a sixty-five-year-old woman runs 400m in well under 70 seconds, or an eighty-year-old woman does so in less than 90 seconds, those are, when you think about them, absolutely breathtaking achievements. But unless you have actually attempted something similar yourself, while familiarising yourself with the norms for different age groups, it's hard to appreciate just how breathtaking. So the neutral observer's attention tends to focus less on what these athletes do than on how they do it. What do they look like as they compete? What do they experience? Does it still feel real – to the athlete or to the spectator? And, more broadly: what drives them on? Are they still functioning more or less as a young person would? And, if not, how has age changed them?

Usually it depends who you ask. One rainy evening, Rietje Dijkman, who would finish the games with four golds, three world records and a European record, was breathtakingly dominant in the W80 100m final, leaving her rivals for dead as casually as Usain Bolt in his prime. How did she do it? Partly with the help of the gym she has set up in the basement of her Amsterdam home; but there was no time to probe: another runner in the race had already distracted me.

Elena Pagu was more than ten seconds slower than Dijkman, finishing the 100m in 27.89 seconds. But she was the one that the local media wanted to interview afterwards, for the simple reason that she was ninety-three, and had just retained her European title, unopposed, in the W90 category. Pagu and Italy's Emma Maria Mazzenga – winner and sole finalist at W85 – had run alongside the W80 finalists, and it was Pagu's finish, the last of seven, that provoked the most excited applause.

She took the attention in her stride. Back in Bucharest, she is a celebrity – one of very few Masters stars to have achieved 'crossover'. She stars in television advertisements, does motivational talks (including a TEDx talk), runs her own vlog, and wears sunglasses to avoid being stopped in the street. When I caught up with her later on, I was bowled over by her charisma. She laughed, twinkled, flirted like a Hollywood grande dame, shrugging off her 100m victory while grumbling furiously about her disqualification earlier in the day in the 5km race walk, at which she used to be world record-holder. She told me about her childhood, climbing cherry trees with her mother ('I asked her: "Is heaven as beautiful as this?"'); and about being wolf-whistled by Soviet soldiers when she walked to school as a teenager; and about her three marriages. She took up running at fifty-seven, to relieve the boredom of unwanted retirement, and scandalised her neighbours by doing so. ('One of them said: "I saw Mrs Pagu running. She went crazy. I saw her with my own eyes ..."') Eight years after that, she won her first medal. 'The first time I heard them playing the Romanian anthem, I felt so euphoric I thought I could fly.' She wanted more, and now, at ninety-three, had a whole hallway full of medals in her Bucharest apartment, including six European golds and nine World golds.

Is she fast? It's hard to judge such things. Her time in

Caorle was arguably slow even for her age group: 27.89 seconds for 100m, compared with a W90 world record of 23.15, set by Japan's Mitsu Morita in 2013. You would expect Mazzenga (21.56 at eighty-six) and Dijkman (17.26 at eighty) to prove considerably faster when their turn comes. But their turn hasn't yet come – that's the point – and who knows what the intervening years will bring? The main challenge at that age is simply to be there: alive, well, active and keen. And happy. Pagu had got those basics right.

The longer she continues to do so, the more exceptional she becomes (she has subsequently set a world record in the W95 category), and the more her stardom brightens. As a widow, she is grateful for the attention. 'The heart', she likes to say, 'does not wrinkle.' But it's the actual act of running that suffuses her being with enthusiasm. 'For me running is not a sport,' she bubbled, grey eyes sparkling. 'It's a way of life.' And while there are still those who tell her that, at her age, she should take things easy, she scorns such advice: 'An old person who has nothing to do is ready to be buried.'

Pagu's passion made a deep impression on me. She was old – very old – yet full of joy. Her face had laughter lines, not wrinkles, and she rarely stopped smiling – as if she were still dreaming in colour. Maybe I could learn to do likewise, I told myself; and when I imagined my own old age in those terms, it began to feel, tentatively, like something I could look forward to.

After the Games, people who know much more about such matters than I do enthused about the achievements of British superstars such as Clare Elms, who won five individual W55 golds (at 1500m, 5,000m, 10,000m, 4km cross-country and 10km road race); Virginia Mitchell, who beat Elms into second place in both the 400m and the 800m; Donald Brown, who won M55 golds at 100m, 200m and 100m hurdles; Ian Richards, who won three individual M70 race-walking golds and would have smashed a world record as well had the 10km road walk course been the correct distance; and Angela Copson – whose imperious victory in the W70 800m took her lifetime tally of European golds to thirteen (along with ten World golds, thirty-six British ones, and so many other medals that she barely has room in the cupboard under her stairs for the shoeboxes she keeps them in). At the time, however, many of these achievements barely registered with me. Instead, my gaze kept drifting to the oldest athletes: the ones who were running out of time.

There was, for example, a remarkable relay race. It involved a team of elderly Germans, with a combined age of 346 years, who had set their hearts on an M85 world record in the 4x400m. Their attempt was hardly fast: they were outside the 'real' (non-Masters) world record after a lap and a half. But it was a triumph of age management by their team leader, Herbert Müller.

A seemingly indestructible eighty-nine-year-old from Grevenbroich, near Dusseldorf, Müller had already won three individual golds at these championships (at 200m, 400m and 800m), despite being at the wrong end of his five-year age group. But he loves running 400m (unlike most older runners) and had noticed that the existing relay record was soft. All he needed was three other Germans aged eighty-five or over who were able and willing to race with him. This required months of careful searching and persuasion, but eventually Müller's efforts (later celebrated in a big article in *Die Zeit*) produced a just-about-viable team. Edi Bscheid – an eighty-seven-year-old former ice hockey player with chronic Achilles problems – was persuaded to drop out of the decathlon, while Armin Zosel, who had even less experience of the distance, switched from the half-marathon. Müller's friend Friedrich Ingenrieth completed the team, despite a dodgy Achilles, a recent brush with thrombosis and a hearty dislike of races of more than 200m.

Other weaknesses in the team included Bscheid's suspect hearing (what if he didn't hear the starting gun?); Müller's limited vision in one eye (risky for baton changes); and Ingenrieth's arthritic right hand (bad for accepting the baton) and weak left hand (worse still for giving it). But careful allocation of the legs limited the risks posed by their various frailties. Unfortunately, there was no time to practise, and although Müller explained the rules to the other three the night before the race, he couldn't be sure that it had sunk in.

On the day, Müller was relieved that they all remembered to turn up at the right time and place. They weren't all wearing the same version of the German strip, but you can't have everything. The race started well: Bscheid heard the starter's pistol. Then, after a few strides, a calf strain reduced him to an agonised limp. Spectators urged him on, but the lap took him well over two minutes, which didn't bode well. Yet the other three had come too far to give up lightly. Müller, wiry as his wire-framed glasses, ran a heroic second lap of 1:40 and Zosel managed 1:50 for the third. Ingenrieth began the anchor lap sharply but then he, too, ground to a near-halt. It was the hottest day of the Games – around 30 degrees C – and by the final 100 metres he had slowed to a painful shuffle. Yet he kept going, to his team-mates' loud delight, to complete a world record of 7:23.31.

There were other records set that day, including a world record by the British W55 4x400m relay team (4:27.33 by Julie Rogers, Christine Anthony, Janice Ella-cott and Virginia Mitchell) and a European record by the British W65 team (5:00.12 by Caroline Marler, Rosalind Tabor, Joylyn Saunders-Mullins and Caroline Powell). By any objective standard, these were much more signifi-cant sporting achievements. Yet somehow it was the Germans' ramshackle triumph that caught the public's imagination – because their struggle with the ageing process was much more visible.

In the same way, there was widespread excitement at Giuseppe Ottaviani's triumph in the long jump. You had to watch closely to discern his winning leap at all: it was well under a metre, and looked a bit like a man jogging into a sandpit. But if you watched in the knowledge that Ottaviani was 103, it was a thrilling spectacle; especially if you then thought about some of the other very old peo-ple in your life, and imagined how startled you'd be if one of them suddenly broke into a run or leaped off the ground. Ottaviani did both, six times in all, although four of his jumps were fouls. His winning jump (0.65m) was well short of his European record (1.33m, set just after turning 100), but it was unbeatable for gold medal purposes: there was no one else in his age category.

Afterwards, athletes, officials and spectators queued up for selfies with him. He was happy to oblige but kept being distracted by journalists – and clearly relished both kinds of attention. A former tailor from Sant'Ippolito in the Marche region, he was small, restless and talkative, with none of the tentativeness or timidity that the physically frail often reveal in their mannerisms. 'Without effort, life isn't much,' he declared after collecting his medal, the sinking sun glinting from his spectacles. 'Sport is good for health, for happiness, for friendship. Sport is life, and every day should be lived to the full.'

Italy's media was there in force to watch him do so. The nation had barely finished mourning its other grand old man of track and field, the sprinter, author, entrepreneur and Coca-Cola advertising icon Ugo Sansonetti, who had died in Rome, aged 100, a few weeks earlier. So perhaps they were more than usually aware of a crucial rule with very old athletes: you need to enjoy them while you can. This was certainly true of Ottaviani. He died peacefully nine months later, soon after his 104th birthday: an unsurprising development that none the less adds poignancy to his final moments of sporting glory.

But transience is an occupational hazard for Masters athletes, whatever their age. Every competitor at the Games was just one bad injury away from ceasing to be an athlete; and when that happened, further decline would follow. Most of them knew this. But those who had been around the longest seemed to feel it most intensely. 'We like to make the most of each day,' said Slávka Ročnáková, winner of the W70 steeplechase, 'because tomorrow it could all be snatched away.' She smiled fondly across the café table at her ninety-year-old husband, Karel Matzner, who won silvers in the M90 400m and 800m and bronze at 200m. They had just showed me their sizeable medal collection, and it was clear that they took results and records as seriously as anyone. Matzner was a founding father of the Czech veteran athletics association, whose story he once told in a book; and he and Ročnáková had spent decades on the association's committees. I'm afraid I couldn't tell you anything more specific about their sporting achievements (although I do have them written down somewhere). What I do remember, vividly, is how, all the time we were talking, they couldn't stop smiling at one another.

'The secret,' said Matzner, 'is to find the joy in sport. A positive mental attitude helps you keep running, and running helps you have a positive mental attitude.' They hadn't missed a major championship since 1991, said Ročnáková, even when Matzner, then eighty-seven, had injured himself badly falling off a ladder just before the 2016 World Championships in Australia. 'He couldn't run, but I took him with me anyway,' said Ročnáková. 'It was better than leaving him alone at home.'

'You have to find the joy today,' said Matzner, 'because we don't know what awaits us.'

You could argue that, in fact, the oldest athletes know exactly what awaits them: they're near the top of Death's 'to do' list. (He finally got round to the much-loved Matzner in November 2021.) Yet perhaps for that very reason the old Masters fiercely resist any attempt to limit their lives with conventional thinking about old people's frailty. Vanessa Hannam, an Australian-born foster carer from Kent who was representing Great Britain in the W45 javelin, discus and shot put, told me how, on a day when she wasn't competing, she took a bus trip to see Venice. On the return journey, the bus was crowded, so she offered her seat to a pale old German man with thin white hair and a rather skeletal face. He refused indignantly. 'He got quite cross. He said: "I won a gold medal in the over-eighties 100 metres yesterday!"'

Every athlete at the Games would recognise that defiance. The very act of competing affirms your identity as someone who is still a fully functioning human being; a medal does so with added emphasis. It's like saying to the world, 'Other people may be old. I'm normal.'

Even in the younger Masters age groups, athletic competition can offer powerful validation of your identity as a human individual – unlimited by non-youthful labels such as 'parent' or 'spouse'. Hannam, who won bronze in the javelin and came fourth in the discus and shot put, came to Masters athletics via a relatively common route, re-starting in mid-life. She excelled at her events in her teens, took a twenty-seven-year break for migration, marriage and motherhood, then recently made space for a little more 'me' in her life. 'I thought, maybe I should try throwing again, to see if I can still do it' – and before she knew it she had a European medal.

John Wright, by contrast, had been a complete novice when he turned to running in his forties; but he too had made the shift from parent to protagonist. 'I was taking my daughter to athletics and I thought: "I'll give this a try."' Now the Chorley athlete was an M60, with years of ferocious training behind him, and had just won three emphatic golds in the sprints. There was still something dad-like about him – receding hair, glasses, greying beard, a thoughtful manner – but plenty of runners half his age would envy his powerful physique and, in many cases, his winning times: 12.3 seconds for 100m, 25.6 seconds for 200m and 58.6 seconds for 400m. He knows that the wheels will come off one day, but competes all the more fiercely for that. 'We don't just come here to have fun,' he told me. 'Everyone wants to win.'

Perhaps he was right. But winning takes many forms. Only an elite minority of international Masters competitors can realistically hope for a medal. But all can hope for a triumph of some kind: a performance they're proud of, a landmark they've been aiming for; or the simple achievement of competing with the best, at an international championship, at an age when it would be much easier not to do so.

This sank in for me at an event that had nothing to do with the track. It took place towards the end of the Games in a big, neon-lit nightclub on the outskirts of Jesolo, where the organisers had arranged a party for athletes, officials and volunteers. There was a Fifties theme, with music by Les Babettes and Mr Wallace All Stars, and I was patronisingly expecting a 'pensioners' disco'. But it didn't feel like that at all.

The venue shone with twenty-first-century bling, with palm trees and a swimming pool and what looked like Perspex ceiling tiles, and an eye-wateringly expensive bar – which may or may not have had a bearing on my observation that Masters athletes drink sparingly. What they don't do sparingly is dance. The music turned out to span many genres and periods – although not the twenty-first century – and the dance floor heaved from early on with fit, tanned bodies, swaying to the rhythms of teenage years gone by. Some dressed in keeping with the Fifties dress code; others had chosen outfits evoking their own youthful tastes in subsequent or preceding decades.

The result was a patchwork of conflicting styles, musical and sartorial, held together by a general shininess and a raw physical energy that felt disconcertingly adolescent. The night wore on. The sense of exuberance intensified. You could almost feel the wild lust for life. Smiles flashed, eyes sparked, silver hair gleamed; satin jackets glittered in the violet light. 'Blue Suede Shoes' gave way to 'Tie A Yellow Ribbon', then slowed to 'Can't Help Falling in Love'. Bodies swayed closer, some with the poignant tenderness of decades-old romance and some with what looked more like speculative sexual opportunism. Both felt strangely transgressive. Old people aren't supposed to experience life in such ways – are they?

Then it struck me: this was the whole point. That was why these people had come to Italy for this strange, vigorous Club 35–103 holiday: because they refused to accept the limitations their age is supposed to impose on them. They wanted to carry on feeling fully alive.

Were they rebels? Perhaps. Or maybe they just didn't realise that they were old. Either way, there was clearly a whole spectrum of activities on which they were determined not to give up: not just competitive sport but sex, romance, partying, travelling, dancing, starting each day in hope, laughing noisily, making new friends, discovering new adventures. Whatever their age, they had decided to carry on living.

And, just as the wiser ones had learnt to run each race as if it might be their last, so the athletics habit seemed to have taught many of these Masters to live each day with the same perspective, giving thanks for each fast-vanishing moment. It would be hard to think of a better formula for feeling intensely and colourfully alive; and it showed.

I left Caorle full of envy. I had looked into the Gold Zone, and I liked what I saw. But it felt very much like their zone, not mine: a world within a world in which a gifted few brightened the experience of ageing through competitive athletics. There wasn't any point, was there, in an out-of-shape, injury-prone jogger like me kidding myself that I might one day join them?

Yet in the weeks that followed I couldn't let go of that thought. It would obviously be out of the question for the immediate future: the Masters athletes in my age group were way out of my league, even if I did manage to get back into my running groove. But perhaps at some point in the distant future, in one of those older age categories, it would be something to explore.

First, though, I needed to solve a more fundamental problem: how to keep going as a runner at all.

6

Urban legends

I recognised Ginette Bedard's house from the medals dangling in the porch. Apart from that, there wasn't much to distinguish it from all the other small, square, weatherboarded, neat-lawned houses in the gusty grid of near identical streets known as Howard Beach, in the shadow of John F. Kennedy International Airport. Luckily, she was in.

That hadn't been a given, because Ginette is often out. You can see her out on the waterfront most mornings. You can see her most afternoons, too, if you happen to be looking in the right place. She's the one running: a stooping figure in a bright bandana. She's usually out there for three hours a day. If she isn't, it might be because she's racing, possibly in a marathon.

She seemed like a good person to meet. She'll be eighty-nine by the time you read this, if she's spared, and she had been featuring for years in reports of the New York City Marathon, invariably tagged as the oldest runner in the race. So I figured that she must know something about staying power, not just in the sense of keeping going for miles and miles but in the more important sense of keeping going for years and years.

She was happy to talk to me, and delighted that I shared her enthusiasm for running. But if she had a secret, she had no idea what it was. Speaking loudly and rapidly, with extravagant hand gestures, she told me that she grew up on a farm near Metz, in the Lorraine region of France. She was active but not sporty. When she was twenty-two she met a Canadian airman, Gerald Bedard, on a local dance floor, 'and la-la-la, one thing led to another.' They married, moved to Canada and then, seven years later, relocated to Howard Beach, New York.

She liked it there. It's an unfashionable corner of Queens, but there's room to breathe, even if the air does sometimes taste of aviation exhaust. Their little red-brick house, where Ginette still lives, is just a couple of blocks from the windswept waterfront on Jamaica Bay. The air-craft noise wasn't too overwhelming then, in the early 1960s, and the nearby salt-water wetlands of Hawtree Creek and Shellbank Basin were rich with wildlife. As for work, it couldn't have been handier for Gerald, and Ginette soon found her own job at the airport, too. For more than thirty years she worked on the Alitalia cus-tomer service desk, where her cheerful, energetic nature and winning smile made up for her still imperfect mas-tery of English. She also raised two children – one of whom found long-term employment of her own at JFK.

There wasn't much space in Ginette's life for sport, but she kept herself in shape, mainly by following the TV workouts of the fitness guru Jack LaLanne. Only when retirement was looming did it occur to her that she might – like countless other New Yorkers in the late 1990s – become a runner. Gerald tried it first; then Ginette, tentatively, did a bit of jogging of her own, along the nearby waterfront. 'I had to get up at 3.30 a.m., so that I'd be finished in time to go to work.' Then a colleague at Alitalia mentioned that he had done a marathon. 'At first I thought, people who do that must be superhuman. But later I thought, if he can do it, why can't I?'

In 2001, aged sixty-eight, she joined New York Road Runners – 'the best thing I ever did' – and started racing at distances from a mile to 10k. In 2002, nine months short of her seventieth birthday, she ran her first New York City Marathon. Her time, 4:15:55, would have been respectable for a beginner of any age.

Apart from 2012 and 2020, when it wasn't run, and 2021, when it was run in reduced form, she has run the NYC Marathon every year since, along with a smattering of other marathons and hundreds of races at shorter distances. Her best times over 26.2 miles were 3:46:34 in the NYC Marathon in 2005; 3:46:03 in the More Marathon (also in New York City) in 2006, which was a US record for a woman in her seventies; and 4:08:31 in the NYC Marathon in 2008, which was (briefly) a world record for a woman over seventy-five. Her slowest was 7:39:08 in 2019, aged eighty-six, although with luck she'll keep going long enough to do even slower ones. What makes her a local legend is not her speed – her records have already been broken – but her cheerful, indomitable persistence.

Since 2014 she's been a member of the USA Track & Field Masters Hall of Fame, and for New York Road Runners she's something between an icon and a mascot, constantly honoured at club nights. She posed for the *New York Times* magazine in her swimsuit – aged eighty-one. The *New Yorker* made a short film about her, and she has featured in many TV interviews. She has so many medals, trophies, plaques, statuettes and framed photos and certificates that there's barely room for her trainers in the office-cum-porch where she keeps them. For the wider public, the later stages of the NYC Marathon simply wouldn't be the same without her flamboyant presence. She loves the attention.

At races, she is a distinctive figure, recognisable by her bright bandanas, and by her plentiful make-up, which sometimes runs when she does. Her rationale is that 'I don't want to look like an old bag' when photographed, but it sometimes seems to be more than that: lavish lipstick and eyeshadow flaunted as a cheerful two fingers to the whole tiresome idea of growing old. She once tried running in her big blonde wig, for similar reasons, but it kept slipping, so she leaves it at home now. Either way, the younger runners love her, and she is always ready with a smile and some uplifting words for anyone who asks.

But no one reaches their late eighties without suffering. Her children grew up and moved on. Her life began to empty. Friends died or moved. Gerald, eight years older than her, developed dementia. In 2015 he died, aged eighty-nine. 'It was very sad,' said Ginette. 'I miss him. It was *la merde*. I ran to keep myself sane. I ran before, and during, and after.'

Even now, she uses running as a lifeline. 'I run ten miles a day. It's wonderful. If I only run seven or eight miles, I come back depressed. If I do my ten miles, I come back happy.' That's the nearest thing she has to a formula. The older she gets, the longer it takes, so she does half her running first thing in the morning, after a coffee and a slice of brioche, and the rest towards the end of the afternoon. Each session takes about an hour and a half. 'That's normal. When you get older, you get slower.'

She eats 'in moderation' but is far from picky: wine,

cheese and ice cream all play a part in her diet. As for other exercise, she does a little bit of stretching most days, and usually a few press-ups, but otherwise she just runs: ninety minutes in the morning, ninety in the afternoon, come rain or shine, every day of the year apart from race days.

She always trains on the same route, up and down the waterfront, overlooking the airport end of Jamaica Bay. It's a bleak place, or a wild, bracing one, depending on your mood. The Atlantic wind scythes in from beyond Rockaway, its whoosh blending with the rumble of the jets above and the traffic on Cross Bay Boulevard. Ducks and Canada geese drift on the grey water, or peck moodily on land, scattering at a jogger's approach. That's what they did when I tried it, anyway. When Ginette approaches, they rush to meet her. 'They love me. I bring them sunflower seeds. I love my duckies.'

Sometimes she runs on the sand; mostly she runs on the largely traffic-free tarmac: backwards and forwards, slightly hunched, taking short, fast, busy, slightly jerky steps. When she races, her face sometimes seems clenched with grim resolve. When she trains, her head is empty. 'I don't think about much,' she said. 'I see aeroplanes flying by. I see my duckies. But I never come back sorry. You're only sad when you don't do it.'

It's a phrase she often repeats: *you never come back sorry*. Most runners will know what she's getting at. Running doesn't solve her problems, but it makes it easier to face them bravely. 'I'm lonely,' she admitted. 'I need a boyfriend. But the guys my age are kaput, and the younger ones are all married, like you.' (She had already enquired about this.) She was simultaneously joking and bitterly serious. This is what happens when you hang on to your youthful health for longer than your contemporaries. You lose them – and what do you do after that?

'The problem isn't feeling old. I feel like I'm thirty-six. The trouble is looking old. There's nothing wrong with me. I can still wear the bikini I had when I was sixteen. But the wrinkles . . .'

Ginette would like to find a partner: someone who could share her love of running, at least to some degree. 'But who the hell still runs at my age?' Instead, she suspects, fellow octogenarians feel threatened by her fitness and energy, while anyone younger would be likely to think her freakish. An old woman who runs? No, that's weird. From Ginette's perspective, however, it's her convention-bound contemporaries whose lives have gone off track: at least she's still living hers. 'People tell me: "I used to be—." Well, I "used to be" too. But I still am.'

Meanwhile, social prejudice against the 'over-active' old is just one more reason to keep on running. Among her 'running family' at New York Road Runners, Ginette is accepted for what she is, and can mingle without awkwardness with other age groups. (That's one of the beauties of running clubs generally.) But in any case, she would never slow down just to conform to her neighbours' expectations. Running is what keeps her sane.

'I'll never stop running,' she insisted. 'Not until I drop dead.'

That's my plan too, I told her. I'm just struggling to stick to it, which is why I came to her for her tips. But her guidance is minimalist. 'Just keep running,' she laughed. 'You get out what you put in. If you keep running every day like me, you can run until you're a hundred.'

*

I left Ginette's house feeling full of hope and enthusiasm. Yet I didn't feel much the wiser about how she had been able to sustain her running habit. Was it attitude? Luck? Or some other quality?

A few weeks later, back in the UK, I got in touch with Ken Jones. He is three months older than Ginette but has been running for much longer; and, like her, makes regular headlines as the oldest competitor in a major big city race. In his case, it's the London Marathon, which – the first time I spoke to him – he had just run for the fortieth year in a row.

He had had to run it virtually that time, up and down a deserted lane near his home near Strabane, Northern Ireland; but it was enough to ensure continued membership of the 'Ever Presents', an exclusive band who have completed every London Marathon since it was founded in 1981. There were forty-two such runners when the group was first identified in 1995, but by 2020 it had just ten members, and by 2021 just seven, of whom Ken was the oldest.

He hadn't particularly enjoyed his virtual race, apart from the supportive company of his daughter, Heather, who ran the whole distance with him. He missed the buzz of the physical event: the shared journeys with younger runners, the reunions with old friends. But the worst thing had been the rain. 'It was the worst weather I've ever run in,' he said, 'and I've done thousands of races. It wasn't just pouring. It was torrential. I've never known anything like it.' The pair had planned to start at 9 a.m. but delayed it by an hour, and then by another hour, in the hope that the deluge would ease. It didn't: it just grew windier. When they finally started, Ken wore a thick raincoat, plus thermal top, lightweight vest and lined leggings, but they had to stop three times to change into drier clothing. They even tried running with an umbrella for a while, although this proved too awkward to sustain. After 18 miles Ken felt ready to quit – but he was old enough to know better. 'I've been there before many times, so when this feeling comes along, it hits you in the head, but I know I have to beat it.' So he just kept on plugging away, alternating between jogging and a fast walk, trying not to focus on the discomfort. He knew that he would never forgive himself if he stopped. 'I just wanted that medal. You could have dug ditches in front of me, or built walls, and I'd have just climbed over. I'd have run through hell to get it.'

He and Heather eventually completed the distance in just under eight hours: 7:53:34, to be precise. Perhaps he felt a flicker of disappointment when he saw the time. Once, he had been able to run a marathon almost three times as fast. But any such pang would have been quickly overwhelmed by waves of relief and satisfaction. It was pitch dark, and the rain had only just begun to ease to a drizzle. A few neighbours – masked, of course, against Covid – had braved the wet night to clap him home. And then – well, anyone who has ever run a marathon can imagine the happiness. He was soon warm and dry; Heather was cooking him bubble and squeak; he could put his feet up; and he could bask in the thrilling glow of a major achievement accomplished – the kind of glow that very few octogenarians get the chance to enjoy.

He had already put his name down for the next year's race – even before sinking gratefully into his bed and dissolving into well-earned sleep. 'You've got to have a target,' he explained. Like Ginette, he instinctively looks forward, not back. But when I did persuade him to reminisce, it was not immediately obvious what else they had in common.

Unlike Ginette, Ken has been running for most of his life, mainly in England, where he lived until 2003. Born in Wembley, in the shadow of the stadium, he left school at thirteen ('I could barely read or write') and spent much of his early life as a dockyard labourer in Chatham, Kent. National service took him to West Germany, where he discovered competitive running. Eventually, in the early 1960s, he married, settled down in Chingford, and became a policeman – first a bobby on the beat, then a traffic officer and eventually a crime investigation officer. Soon he was running for the Metropolitan Police, at anything from 5 to 20 miles. Then, in 1963, he joined Orion Harriers and began to concentrate on cross-country. Epping Forest, a short warm-up jog from his front door, was the perfect training ground: 'It was beautiful, and so interesting, with lovely horse-rides to run on, and little streams everywhere, and hills and ponds. It was the perfect running place. I ran there every day. I knew every inch of it.'

He was thirty-four when he first raced over 26.2 miles, and although his debut was unspectacular, he felt that the longer distance suited him. He began to run marathons regularly – his best time was 2:41 in the Polytechnic Marathon in Middlesex – and by the time the first London Marathon was held in 1981, forty-eight-year-old Ken had about forty of them under his belt. He came back in 1982, and in 1983, and before he knew it it had become a habit, which in turn became a streak. His best time for London was in 1985, when he ran 2:55, a few weeks before his fifty-second birthday. His toughest race was the following year, when he slipped on a wet manhole cover and hit his head on the pavement. Badly dazed, he was helped into an ambulance before deciding to get out and complete the race.

After that, it would have seemed feeble not to keep his streak going, even as his life moved through its successive phases. He became a grandfather. He retired, reluctantly and late, from the police force. ('I hadn't had a day's illness for fifteen years.') He exchanged Epping Forest for the unfamiliar lanes around Strabane, where his wife, Nora, had family. ('The fields are full of cows, so I run in the lanes.') He became a great-grandfather. Later, Nora's health began to fail, and the bleak likelihood arose that, in due course, he would become a widower.

Through all these life stages, he kept on returning to the London Marathon, April after April, and the joy of catching up with his fellow Ever-Presents steadily became a more important part of the excursions. In Strabane, meanwhile, new friendships blossomed, with local runners of many ages, some of whom shared his enthusiasm for an annual marathon in London. 'I've made hundreds of friends through running,' says Ken. He's too modest to say that he has fans all over Strabane, but he does. Some of them even braved the weather to cheer him on for part of his virtual marathon; and when the Olympics came to London in 2012, Ken was chosen to carry the Olympic Torch through the streets of his adopted town.

He is almost ninety now but still wears his age lightly. He's a small man (about 5ft 9in), with pink cheeks, sparse white hair and a warm, gap-toothed smile. If it weren't for a slight resemblance to a house elf – a facial disproportion that affects most older men, as the ears and nose keep growing long after everything else has stopped – you would think he was in his seventies. But 2020 had been a tougher year than most. Nora died, after sixty years of marriage, and then, while Ken was still in shock, the coronavirus pandemic brought the rest of normal life to a halt. The subsequent isolation was, at times, acute. 'My neighbours look after me,' he told me, gratefully, 'but the pandemic has confined me to the house. I can't go to the shops because I don't want to catch this virus, because that would stop me dead.'

But he kept on running; and while there's running, there's hope. 'I go out first thing in the morning,' he explained during one lockdown, 'when there's no one around.' It was the first time in fifty years that he hadn't gone out at least once a week for a group run, and he was missing it. 'Runners are basically a decent lot of people. You meet them and they give you friendship and keep your life happier.' But even a solitary run was better than nothing. 'If you ever get down in the dumps, you've just got to get yourself together and start training again. You go for a run, you think it over, you're enjoying the views, and you seem somehow to overcome problems. All of a sudden you come back and you feel good.'

I didn't need persuading of any of this. I had already resolved that, if I must grow very old, I would very much like to do so in the active, upbeat style of Ken or Ginette. But Ken's advice on how to follow in his footsteps was scarcely less minimalist than Ginette's. 'Don't stop,' he said simply. 'People tail off around fifty. I have old friends that I used to run with, and they don't run any more. They've got knee trouble, or they've put on weight and got a big belly. If you stop, it's very hard to start again. So

I always try to do something. And if I have a day where I just don't want to do anything, I'll at least walk up to the top of the hill and back again. Even a little is better than nothing.'

Apart from that, it's common sense. He avoids alcohol, tobacco, caffeine and sweet foods; eats simple, nutritious meals (porridge, soup, shepherd's pie); keeps a vague but not obsessive eye on his weight (he's a stone-and-a-half heavier than in his racing prime); and regularly reminds himself to enjoy his running.

A typical training week might include four long, brisk walks along country lanes, often incorporating jogging but always with half an eye on the scenery and wildlife; and (lockdowns permitting) three half-hour sessions at the local swimming pool. So it isn't intense; and he keeps high-impact activities to a minimum. 'But when the training's done I'm always active afterwards, doing house-work or working in the garden.'

He also does a few t'ai chi exercises for his arms and legs, plus some bending to stretch his lower back, and, most impressively, a four-minute 'plank' session (elbows and toes on the floor, body and legs straight and rigid) every morning. He wears compression socks, too – 'I wish they'd invented them years ago' – and makes a point of looking after his feet. ('You need to keep an eye on your toenails.') Otherwise, though, it's just a question of keeping going.

He still feels the weight of his age, sometimes. 'I've been running for seventy years. My body's telling me to stop.' He has to train for two or three hours for the benefit he used to get in sixty minutes, and his marathon time gets slower each year. But he remains injury-free, which is a huge advantage. 'Apart from that time when I hurt my head in the marathon, I've never really had any serious injuries.' Perhaps he's just lucky; but, he pointed out, he has consistently resisted the temptation to over-train. 'Now and again, when I have a race, you have to pull your finger out and push yourself. But with training you mustn't overdo it.'

It sounds disappointingly tame, but it has brought him one big prize: he has continued to run, without significant interruption. As a result, he continues to enjoy the general health benefits that a running habit tends to bring. It's a virtuous circle: he can run because he does run. 'There's nothing really wrong with my body,' he boasted. 'Thanks to running, I'm healthy and fit. Illnesses come knocking at my door, but they don't get in. I feel like a young man.'

They say that the secret of a long marriage is not to get divorced. Perhaps the secret of life-long running is equally simple: don't stop. Keep on running – even if you sometimes have to stop temporarily and start again; even if you keep on getting slower; even if you sometimes have to walk and jog. Just keep putting one foot in front of the other, for however long it takes, and then do it again tomorrow. Some days will be harder than others. But you never come back sorry.

It sounds persuasive. Anyone who has been running for a few years will agree with that. For some of us, however, the formula becomes less effective as we age. The stopping becomes too easy; the starting again too difficult. We'd like to keep on running, but something prevents us from doing so.

And something else allows the lucky few to dodge that something.

7

The grey tradition

For most of human history, no one gave much thought to what runners could or couldn't do in later life, for the good reason that few people lived much beyond forty. You started slowing down as you hit your thirties, and if hunger or disease didn't then get you, foes or predators would.

Over the past two centuries, however, medical, technological and social progress have made loss of fighting fitness increasingly survivable. Average lifespans have doubled, and our sense of what is 'normal' has evolved in response.

The official redrawing of late life's conceptual borders began in the English-speaking world in the late nineteenth century, when a succession of judicial rulings and Acts of Parliament in the UK included definitions of old age as 'not under fifty' or 'any age after fifty'. Then, in the early twentieth century (1908 in the UK), the state started footing the bill for old age pensions, and the threshold was hastily shunted up to seventy. In due course, when the world wasn't at war, average lifespans crept up to match.

Perceptions of normality in sport evolved in parallel. Nineteenth-century headlines of the 'Is this Britain's oldest athlete?' variety tended to involve men – Charlie Pearce of Newport Pagnell or W. Dales of Edinburgh, or, before them, pedestrians such as Josiah Heaton or George Wilson – who were barely out of their forties. By the 1920s, on the other hand, a runner needed to be well into his sixth decade to make headlines – as W. H. Grindley did in 1928 when he ran the Liverpool marathon as a fifty-nine-year-old.

Sporting officialdom was slower to adapt. The Boston Marathon, started in 1897, was supposed to represent a new, inclusive kind of racing, and is revered today as the Founding Father of open-to-all-comers big city marathons. Yet when local runner Peter Foley tried to enter the race in 1910, he was barred for being too old. He was fifty-four.

He wasn't a quitter, though. Older runners rarely are. So he shaved off his thick grey beard and raced anyway, starting a minute behind the 169 official runners. By some accounts he ran to a 'continuous ovation' from spectators. He certainly enjoyed himself enough to come back for more, in many subsequent years, all the way into his eighties.

Yet the thinking behind the original rejection persisted. Officialdom wanted running to remain a young person's sport, even in the coming age of longevity. The old just got in the way, except as spectators or administrators – and if those past their prime insisted on donning running vests, who would wear the blazers?

But even the most pigheaded traditionalists cannot turn back the tides of demography. The increase in life-spans had a cause, which was also a symptom: more people were remaining fit and healthy for longer. Some of those people loved sport. Not all were content to be mere spectators.

The century unfolded. What had been unthinkable became merely unusual. Sports fans in many nations read about the breathtaking athletic achievements of, for example, Arthur Newton, a Somerset-born South African farmer who won the first of his five victories in the 54-mile Comrades Marathon when he was thirty-nine and set his final 100-mile world record, in 1934, at the age of fifty-one. Perhaps runners weren't necessarily finished at thirty after all.

Peter Foley, whose idea of training was to walk eight miles into Boston for a beer and then walk home again, ran his final marathon in 1938, aged eighty-two. It was reported to have taken him four-and-a-half hours. But it wasn't official. He started two hours ahead of the field, not a minute behind as he once had, and the thirty-three-year-old winner was within five minutes of catching him. By this time, according to *Time* magazine, Foley was 'gnome-like . . . white-whiskered and toothless'. But he personified a new, alternative vision of sport – further symbolised by the presence in the same race of Clarence DeMar, who came seventh, a few weeks short of his fiftieth birthday. Eight years earlier, in 1930, DeMar, an Olympic medallist, had won the race for the seventh time, aged forty-one. He would still be taking part when he was sixty-five, and by that time the world had changed.

The Veterans Athletic Club, the world's first sports association for the chronologically challenged, was established in the UK in 1931, with the radical proposition that older runners should compete against their own age groups. Its initial impact was limited, but after the Second

World War word spread, especially among fit, youngish men fresh from the armed forces, who had missed out on their best years as competitive athletes. They wanted to see what they could do, ideally in contests where the competition was close enough to bring out the best in them.

This approach to late-life running was slightly different from what had been seen before. A stubborn old-timer like DeMar could keep coming back to his favourite open event, but each year his age left him further off the pace. So he slipped from first in the Boston Marathon to seventy-eighth place. That's a lot of age-related discouragement for one man to absorb without losing motivation. Veterans' athletics offered a more inviting vision of competition: racing against your peers on a level playing field.

It took time to catch on. Every now and then, a new club would appear, in New Zealand, in Germany, or in a British or American region. But participation was limited and local. Then came the 1960s, and the first rumbles of the recreational running boom. Author-coaches such as Arthur Lydiard, Percy Cerutty and Bill Bowerman became best-selling gurus, preaching a gospel of exercise for all, with running, in particular, presented as the key to personal redemption from the otherwise unavoidable horrors of physical decay.

One early disciple of this new creed was David Pain, an Englishman who had settled permanently in San Diego in 1950. By 1965 he was a successful lawyer, forty-three years old, married with four children, with an active lifestyle whose recreations included handball, racquets, surfing, diving, gardening, choral singing – and, since turning forty, running.

The running was just a fitness thing at first. Pain got

into the habit of doing it on his local municipal golf course, the lush and undulating Oceanside Torrey Pines, accompanied by his dog, Suzy. Then, one breezy morning, an angry course official called the police. Pain was apprehended, Suzy bit one of the officers; man and dog were locked up. Released on bail, Pain contacted the San Diego *Evening Tribune*, which ran a big story about the pair of them. The subsequent media furore transformed the case, somewhat disingenuously, into a test case of the free-born American's right to jog, even in middle age.

This was a social and sporting turning point. Here was a runner in his forties who defied the stereotype of the older runner as a freak. He was a confident, successful lawyer, a family man, a pillar of his community who just happened to love running. By the time Pain won his case, like-minded souls had reached out to him from all over America, and Suzy was just one running companion among many.

Being competitive by nature, Pain began to organise occasional 'Masters Miles' for his new friends: the first was held in June 1966, as part of the San Diego Invitational meet at the city's Balboa Stadium. Word spread, and Masters Miles for the over-forties began to crop up at other meets. A new market, running boomers, was discovering a new product: organised athletics for the no-longer-young.

In July 1968 Pain held what he called, rather hopefully, the '1st annual US Masters Track & Field Championships', a two-day event in the Balboa Stadium for over-forties only. Nearly 350 athletes turned up. Many were remarkably good; more importantly, everyone seemed thrilled to be taking part. So there was a next time, and a time after that, and each year standards and numbers rose.

There was interest from overseas, too, which eventually prompted Pain in 1972 to take a squad of US veterans to compete against their peers in Europe. This was a hair-raising experience, involving five countries, six cities, ten days of competition, more than 100 US veterans, large parties of Australians and Canadians, scores of enthusiastic Europeans, and more welcome and farewell parties than was strictly prudent for an excitable gang of travelling runners aged between forty and eighty-seven. But it was a valuable learning experience for all involved – not least for St John's Ambulance in London, who had been convinced that a two-day meet at Crystal Palace was a geriatric health catastrophe waiting to happen but ended up with nothing to treat but blisters.

By the time the tourists went home, a loose consensus had developed about what the future of veteran athletics might look like. Pain's earliest championships had been flawed, with too few age categories (just 40–49, 50–59 and 60+), too few events (triple jump, pole vault, hammer and steeplechase were all omitted) and too few genders (men only). But these misjudgements were quickly acknowledged and corrected, and the revised formula, with five-year age-bands and a full range of events for men and women, seemed to offer the perfect balance of feasibility, credibility and excitement.

Given the depth of talent and enthusiasm that his tour had revealed internationally, it wasn't surprising that Pain (who may also have been the first person to organise a competitive triathlon, although that's a different story) went on to be one of the prime movers behind the inaugural World Masters Track and Field Championships, held in Toronto in 1975. More than 1,400 athletes, from thirty-two nations, were represented. Most came from English-speaking nations: the US, the UK, Australia, New Zealand, Canada, South Africa. But the event was broad enough to set a bigger bandwagon rolling. By 1977, when the second world championships were held in Gothenburg, Sweden, there were forty-five nations involved (and more than 2,600 athletes), and the Masters movement was sufficiently global to justify the creation of the World Association of Veteran Athletes (WAVA), which was later rebranded as World Masters Athletics (WMA).

The subsequent success of the Masters vision makes it easy to forget how 'seat of our pants' (Pain's words) its early manifestations were. But Pain and his collaborators had, in effect, created something rather big from nothing. There had been older runners before, and groups of older runners, and groups of older runners who organised their own competitive events. But this was a comprehensive programme of athletics for (initially) the over-forties, which worked to such widespread satisfaction that it has remained the basic blueprint for all Masters competition since.

There have been modifications, from time to time, and setbacks and set-tos; but the general direction of travel has been forward. The development of age-graded tables, from 1989 onwards, has allowed participants to rate their performances fairly precisely relative to norms and records for their age and gender. The gist, if you're new to this concept, is that 100 per cent represents the world record for that event and age group, and any given performance can be given a percentage score relative to that. Record-breaking performances are by definition over

100, and the tables are in due course adjusted to take them into account. It's an imperfect system, obviously, since it cannot reflect records that have yet to be set; but the sport is more watchable because of it, and more motivating for participants, because it reveals at a glance how well each athlete is doing in the core struggle with age.

Processes for the verification of ages and the ratification of records have also been formalised, and there have been age-related modifications to certain events, such as the 'long' hurdles. Mainly, however, the Masters story has been one of unbroken growth. The big international championships reached saturation point long ago, typically with around 8,000 to 9,000 participating athletes. The WMA's biennial World Masters Athletics Championships have been joined by biennial regional championships and biennial world and regional indoor championships, giving everyone at least two major international championships a year. There's also a whole parallel calendar of World (and regional) Masters Games, organised by the International Masters Games Association, in which athletics is just one sport among several dozen; and in the US, there's also a thriving Senior Olympics movement, organised state by state. To keep things simple, I am using 'Masters' loosely to embrace all these brands. (For serious athletes in Europe, 'senior' tends to mean eighteen-to-thirty-four rather than thirty-five-plus.)

Some people sense that, after half a century, David Pain's one-size-fits-all Masters template might be due for a rethink. That name, for a start. Can we really not come up with something more inclusive than 'Masters'? And then there are the tensions between opposite ends of the late-life athletics spectrum. Are today's perfectly conditioned thirty-five-year-olds, fresh from the Olympics, really wrestling with the same sporting challenges as athletes in their eighties and nineties, many of whom are relatively new to competitive sport?

Somehow, for now, the sport accommodates both extremes, but this can make it unwieldy, especially in the absence of qualifying standards at major championships – where innumerable heats are often needed to weed out no-hopers. 'You get to the point where races have to start at nine in the morning or even earlier but are still going on in some cases at nine o'clock at night,' says Arthur Kimber, eighty-five-year-old president of the British Masters Athletic Federation (BMAF). But openness to all is a core Masters value.

One day, I suspect, the movement as currently constituted may start to fall apart under the weight of its own success. There's a demographic wave coming, and something will have to give. Maybe there will be streaming for big championships, with no-hopers diverted into secondary events (although their entry fees would be missed), or the sport may be divided by age. Neither idea is popular, but in 2021 and 2022 the British Masters Outdoor Track and Field Championships were split into separate days, one for the thirty-five-to-fifty-four-year-olds and one for the over-fifty-fives. Originally a response to coronavirus, this may or may not become a long-term arrangement.

For the time being, the sport muddles on, partly because only a small minority of runners in their thirties and forties who could identify as Masters choose to do so. What eventually spurs a few of them to make the switch – which in the UK means joining a Masters Area Club that's part of the BMAF – is the chance to compete formally against the best in their age group. But those few are just a drop in the ocean of runners over thirty-five: even before coronavirus, there were fewer than 6,000 British athletes who had signed up to BMAF clubs. The remainder presumably prefer to go on thinking of themselves as 'runners' rather than 'older runners'.

Perhaps that's a good thing, in practical terms. But many Masters yearn for wider recognition, and for more enthusiastic acceptance. Currently, the public accepts that many middle-aged people like to run – which wasn't always the case. ('When I started running as a veteran as a forty-year-old,' says Kimber, 'people used to laugh. Teenagers would shout "Hello, grandad!" – that sort of thing.') But the pensioner who runs too intensely or competitively still risks provoking either laughter or unease. Society tolerates the general idea of Masters athletics, on the basis that it takes all sorts to make a world, and the participants appear to thrive on all that physical activity. But that's very different from valuing the sport as the athletes themselves do.

You have only to compare Masters to the Paralympics – a globally recognised brand – to notice what's missing; or you can visit a major championship. In Masters, such events are still funded by the competitors themselves, via entrance fees. Television is pointedly absent; so are sponsors. Who wants their brand to be associated with the elderly?

In fact, there was a short period, getting on for a decade ago, when the movement almost hit the big time. Two Masters races were included as exhibition events in the World Athletics Championships in Beijing in 2015, allowing fifty-year-olds such as Britain's David Heath (who won gold in the 800m) and Sally Read-Cayton and Virginia Mitchell (gold and silver respectively at 400m) to demonstrate their remarkable speed and endurance to a global television audience. The experiment was repeated the following year at the World Indoor Athletics Championships in Portland, Oregon, where British fifty-two-year-old David Roy Wilcox won gold in the 800m. But then, amid rumours that some administrators considered the Masters a nuisance, the enthusiasm fizzled out.

Today, the vast majority of Masters athletes chase their dreams in obscurity. There are one or two corners of the Masters world – the US road-racing scene, for example – where the very best runners can win significant prize money, but that's very much the exception. In the wider world, the prevailing view – when there is one – remains dismissive. Masters athletics is seen (in the scornful words of German sociologist Henning Eichberg) as 'a true copy of Olympic sport, after the premises of youth, only at a lower level of achievement'. In other words, it's an indulgence.

Serious Masters insist that their sport deserves better than that, not for the sake of their egos but because, if the world doesn't take their sport seriously, potential newcomers can't understand what the sport could offer them. Roger Robinson, the British-born, New Zealand-based author, academic and elite Masters runner, has been arguing for 'parity of respect' for decades. 'When I was first racing Masters, in about 1981, I remember the World Masters Championships in Christchurch, and the media, all they wanted was for someone to fall over the water jump, or for somebody to dodder over a hurdle. That really annoyed me. Here I am fronting up against

Antonio Villanueva and Renato De Palmas – they're absolute gunrunners – we're racing at top level, and they're not taking it seriously . . .'

Robinson was new to Masters at the time, after fifteen years as an 'almost good' international cross-country runner, first for England and then for his adopted country, New Zealand. Now an emeritus professor at Victoria University, Wellington, where he has been teaching literature for thirty-five years, he switched to Masters in early middle age. He found that he was good enough to win M40 and M50 world titles at 10km and cross-country and went on to set age group records for the New York and Boston marathons. Knee problems blighted his sixties but, two replacements later, he is once again a decent contender as an octogenarian, with an M80 10km best of 54:11.

Robinson is also the author of twenty books, six of them on running, including the acclaimed *When Running Made History* (2018). Its final chapter describes the coming of age of Masters athletics, through the prism of the 1989 world championships in Eugene, Oregon: 'the first Masters sports event where there was not a single moment of ageist condescension'. The point, he says, is that the athlete who sets a world record at forty or sixty is pushing back the boundaries of human possibility as surely and significantly as an Olympian who sets a world record at twenty. 'It's top-level international sporting competition, period. Not "incredible at that age".'

When you watch Masters athletics in the flesh, close-up, it's hard to argue with that. You see how the magnitude of the challenge forces the athletes to stretch themselves to breaking point, and you realise that, once you factor in the rules of age-limited events, what you're left with is simply sport. You see a ninety-five-year-old heaving and groaning for air after trying to break thirteen seconds for sixty metres, and you think: well, what do you expect? That is what the extremes of sport look like. But the uninvolved public see it differently. They're accepting enough of old people who run to keep fit, but they feel distinctly uneasy about old people who deliberately push themselves to the furthest frontiers of endurable pain.

There is, says Robinson, 'still this sense of – not exactly disapproval, but anxiety: a sense that when you get to my age it's inappropriate to run to the edge of distress.' Specifically, he adds: 'There are two things you get from people. One: it doesn't look good. And the other is: you might be damaging yourself. And I say: those are exactly the two things that they used to tell women in the 1960s.'

This seems like a rash comparison for a man to make, but Robinson is well-placed to make it. He has shared the past three and a half decades of his life with an American wife who is the ultimate embodiment of women's fight for equality in running. You probably know her name. Kathrine Switzer was the first woman to run officially in the Boston Marathon. She did so as a naïve twenty-year-old, in 1967, having registered as 'K. V. Switzer'. Several miles into the race, a furious race director tried to rip off her numbered race bib and drag her from the course – only for Kathrine's then boyfriend to flatten him with a shoulder charge. Switzer, shocked and shaken, forced herself to complete the race, and the next day there were pictures on every front page. The Amateur Athletic Union subsequently changed its rules to explicitly prohibit women from competing against men, but it was too late. Switzer – and the number (261) on her bib – had gone viral. She has championed the cause of women in running ever since. She wrote a best-selling book, *Marathon Woman*; directed the Avon International Women's Running Circuit, whose success led to the belated acceptance (in 1984) of the women's marathon as an Olympic event; and for good measure won the New York City Marathon in 1974. Later, she founded a non-profit organisation, 261 Fearless, that helps women around the world to empower themselves – and loosen centuries-old chains of prejudice and intimidation – through running.

To equate the frustrations of the pensioner-athletes of the developed nations with the plight of the wider world's oppressed female millions is in one sense grotesque. At certain levels, however, the comparison is valid, and when I run her husband's comments past her Switzer responds: 'Bingo! That sums it up perfectly.' In both cases, she argues, being a particular age or sex creates pressure 'to conform to what that category demands. Example: women should strive to be feminine, attractive, obedient. And older people should strive to be settled, content and wise and not try to imitate or live like a young person.'

Switzer, running her first Boston Marathon in 1967, saw female onlookers who 'looked stunned' when they saw her, as if she were 'something unimaginable'. In a sense, she was, because, as she wrote in *Marathon Woman*, the reason many of these women weren't out there racing too was 'because they actually believed all those myths about women's fragility and limitation, and the reason they believed them is because they had no opportunity to experience something else.' There are millions of old people of whom you could say much the same thing. In most cases, it's not so much the fear of violence or sexual assault that keeps them sitting indoors as something more age-specific. Maybe it's a feeling of vulnerability, brought on by unfamiliar experiences of physical frailty. Maybe it's fear of ridicule – the sense that, as Robinson puts it, 'old people venturing into extreme physical effort are only embarrassing'. Or maybe it's a question of not even realising that the possibility of being a pensioner-athlete exists.

And that, argue Masters enthusiasts, is why parity of respect matters. It's about creating a collective sense of late-life possibility.

Noora Ronkainen, whose in-depth research into the mindsets of ageing athletes has taken her from her native Finland to Denmark, the UK, China and, most recently, Switzerland, where she is an assistant professor at the University of Bern, is one of several academics who have drawn attention to the fact that sport is almost invariably framed as 'a project of youth' involving 'constant progress and upward mobility' – whereas 'the dominant script for ageing in Western cultures is that of decline.' When age does come up in discussions of sport, it is almost invariably as a negative thing: 'Athletes are described as being "over the hill"', says Ronkainen, 'or people talk about the "embarrassment" of the athlete who stays in their sport too long.' This is not only discouraging for young runners, whose sense of self-worth often starts to be eroded by age when they're barely in their thirties. It is also deeply unhelpful for older people, who have no obvious 'exemplary narrative' to encourage them through the later stages of their sporting lives – no hint that those chapters might be thrilling – but, instead, a huge weight of well-meaning prejudice to encourage them back indoors.

Robinson and Switzer – two of the most famous old runners in the world – spent much of Wellington's brief lockdown sneaking out surreptitiously for their daily runs, hoping the neighbours wouldn't see. 'They're a lovely middle-aged couple, very kind,' said Robinson. 'But when all this started they said, "Right, we're going to do your shopping for you." I said, "But I can do our shopping." They said, "You're not going anywhere. You're eighty years old . . ." So I had to put on a hoodie when I went out for a run, because I didn't want them to know that I was ambulatory . . .'

Despite such discouragements, it is possible that, in recent years, an 'exemplary narrative' for late-life athletics has been gaining ground, for several reasons. One is that the best Masters have been getting better, especially in younger age groups. Elite athletes, helped by ever more scientific and professional training, are reaching greater heights of achievement in their primes, and their primes, for the same reasons, are lasting longer. Even when they start to slow, they are fast beyond most imaginations. Just look at the achievements of the Kenyan-American, Bernard Lagat — five-time Olympian, silver and bronze Olympic medallist, double world champion, second-fastest 1500m runner of all time, 5,000m Olympic finalist at the age of forty-one, multiple Masters world record-holder and, at the time of writing, US M40 record-holder at every distance from 1500m (3:41.87 at the age of forty) to marathon (2:12:10 at forty-four). Is Lagat embarrassing himself by not knowing when to quit? Of course not. Perhaps the underlying question has changed slightly, from 'How fast can he go?' to 'How long can he keep this up?' But it's hard to see what's second best about a forty-four-year-old coming within forty seconds of the Olympic qualifying time, at what isn't even his specialist distance. Indeed, it is by no means certain that Lagat's greatest sporting moments are behind him.

Meanwhile, from a different direction, ideas about healthy living and healthy, active ageing have been spreading dramatically. Yes, the pool of sedentary people has grown, but so has the pool of relatively active, relatively healthy people in their fifties and sixties. Some are running-boomers who, like me, have passed involuntarily from 'young' to 'old' but don't feel ready to forgo one of their life's great pleasures. Others, including hundreds of thousands who have come to running via parkruns, have decided in middle age to embrace an active future – sometimes in response to perceived failures in bodily health. So there are, one way or another, a lot more people around for whom Masters athletics might feel vaguely relevant.

Partly as a result of those trends, organised Masters athletics may also, very gradually, be becoming more visible. Over the past decade or so, journalists such as Ken Stone (San Diego-based creator of the influential masterstrack.blog), authors such as Amby Burfoot and Gail Kislevitz (also in the US), film-makers such as Jan Tenhaven and Selah Hennessy (in Germany and the UK respectively) and photographers such as Alex Rotas (in the UK) have energetically chronicled and celebrated the exploits of older athletes, enthusing both the general public (up to a point) and the athletes themselves, who have begun to sense that, at long last, their efforts are no longer going entirely unnoticed.

The combined effect of all this coverage has been to show that old age is much less limiting than we have been taught to believe. In the words of the Bristol-based Rotas, who has done more than most people to change public preconceptions about late-life sport: 'What these athletes in my photos show is what the ageing human body is really capable of.'

Now seventy-two, Rotas first took an interest in Masters athletics as a sixty-year-old academic, whose studies of visual culture had prompted her to wonder if the media's portrayal of female sportspeople changed as they aged. She searched for images of 'older people in sport' and found only 'these absolutely ghastly images of older people sitting in care homes, slumped in their chairs. That's all you got. The images were moribund. They weren't even joyful care homes. These people had all the life force drained out of them.'

Rotas quit academia, learned to use a camera and, through a long, dogged process of trial and error, became an accomplished photographer, with a self-imposed mission to make life-affirming images of old people being active. For the past decade or so, this has meant following the Masters athletics circuit.

She had her first exhibition in 2012, published her first photographic book two years later, and by 2020 had had so much impact that the World Health Organisation decided to launch its Decade of Healthy Ageing with a huge showing of her work – thirty double-sided display-boards, each 2 metres high, beside Lake Geneva – in May 2020. (Covid, sadly, derailed that plan.)

What makes Rotas's work so powerful is the emphasis she places on the athletes' lived experiences as elderly, active people whose wrinkled faces reveal them as 'empowered, focused, determined and joyful'.

'I want to show the emotion and the liveliness,' she says. 'They're old, but they look wonderful, because they've got life in them.'

Not only that: they are living with intense purpose. When Rotas presented copies of her 2014 book, *Growing Old Competitively*, to the athletes who featured in it, she was surprised by how much it meant to some of them. 'For a lot of these events, the stadium is empty. There was one Estonian thrower – we had no common language, but I sought her out and showed her her picture in the book, and she practically cried. It's because I've been a witness to how awesome she is, and maybe nobody else has . . .'

Some of Rotas's favourite images involve 'women in their seventies and their eighties, leaping over a high jump or a long jump or whatever, and they're just throwing themselves around, and they are completely self-abandoned, in a good way, legs akimbo, absolutely wonderfully unselfconscious . . .' This is a vision of ageing in which the old person isn't limited but liberated – perhaps more so than they have been for years. 'You're travelling to different places. You're making new friends, at a time when people are losing their friends. This is a time of life when your life could be narrowing down, but instead, with Masters athletics, it opens up.' Or, as Roger Robinson puts it, it's about 'being totally engaged with life's journey, not merely lingering in its departure lounge.'

All of which suggests that the Masters message is worth spreading. A century ago, athletes were feared to be putting their lives at risk with their efforts to run a sub-four-minute mile. Women were confidently asserted to be incapable of racing more than 800 metres without collapsing. Both assumptions were wrong, but widely held. Then a tiny, pioneering elite disproved them, and many thousands of lesser runners were empowered.

So it is with age, and the pioneering elite of competitive Masters running. Frederico Fischer, the Brazilian sprinter who in the 1970s helped launch the Masters movement in South America, had been urged to quit running on health grounds a decade earlier. 'You're forty years old ...' they told him. But Fischer ignored the received wisdom and went on to set multiple Masters world records, over several decades, notably in the 100 metres at M90 and M95, and as I write this he is an active 105-year-old.

There may not be a ninety-year-old living who could run 100 metres in 17.53 seconds – Fischer's still unbroken M90 record from 2007. But there are probably lots of ninety-year-olds who would enjoy running 100 metres at *some* speed. Fischer's achievements give them – and us – permission to try.

8

The invisible burden

I'm running on Dartmoor on a wild January morning. High, juggernaut clouds sweep the brown slopes with their ominous, fast-moving shadows, but the sky behind them is a fresh, watery blue. The landscape seems vast: fold after fold of coarse, patchworked moor, rolling in all directions to distant blue-grey horizons. The cropped turf is soft but not slippery. Even the granite boulders, rough with old lichen, are grippy enough to run on.

Any normal person would be drinking all this in, marvelling at nature's rich variety and rejoicing in the privilege of being able to run in such a life-affirming environment. But I'm not. I'm beyond caring.

For the past 9 miles or so I've been trying to keep up with five-time Olympian Jo Pavey and her husband and long-term coach, Gavin. And for the past 8 miles or so I've been embarrassing myself. I'm keenly aware that it's a privilege for me to be out with the couple, but that just makes it worse. I'm staggering on the long uphills. The rough downhills are making me light-headed with stabs of knee pain. Even the flat bits – where Jo has a tendency to accelerate dramatically – are making me nauseous. My lower legs are wobbling, my feet are sliding all over the place, and when I gasp for air my chest seems to have shrunk. The only thing I haven't done is shit myself, and I can't even guarantee that much longer.

I suppose it's not surprising. Jo is one of the finest ever examples of athletic durability. She competed in five successive Olympics – the last of them, in 2016, at the age of forty-two. In 2014, ten months after giving birth to her second child, she became the oldest ever female European champion, winning gold in the 10,000 metres in Zurich just a few weeks before her forty-first birthday. She has a clutch of bronze and silver medals too – Commonwealth, European, World – and, although she doesn't really think of herself as a Masters athlete, holds age group world records for 10,000m (W35) and 5,000m (W40). When she turns fifty in 2023, I wouldn't bet against her claiming more, and perhaps turning up to a Masters championship or two.

She is, in short, an athletic superstar, with a rare gift for shrugging off age, who really doesn't need the additional advantage, today, of being thirteen years younger than me. As for Gavin, he's lived on Dartmoor all his life and skips through the rough terrain as carelessly as a dog; even Jo has to work harder than he does on the most treacherous slopes.

I've begged them beforehand to go easy on me. The sad thing is: they are. Sadder still: it's not just the pace that's hurting me. I've run to exhaustion on Dartmoor many times, but I swear it has never hurt this much, or in so many ways. It never felt this cold before, either. Perhaps I'd feel better if I knew how much longer the ordeal would last, but I have lost track of time and place. All I know is that we're above, and sometimes in, the Dart Valley, north of Ashburton; and that our cars are far away. Jo or Gavin could probably tell me more, but I'm ashamed to ask yet again.

The annoying thing is, I ought to be loving this. Jo and Gavin are fascinating and sympathetic running companions, and here they are in their element. Gavin, who is guiding us, repeatedly tweaks our route to ensure I don't miss out on his favourite scenic spots, and the couple's love of the landscape enriches much of their conversation. At one point, we pause on a grassy slope (near the broad, green path known as Dr Blackall's Drive) where, on a winter's day much like this one, they got engaged.

Parts of our route are familiar to me, too: yes, the stooped, balding trees on this hillside still tilt in the same direction as the bare gorse, just as they did the last time I was here. A sweet, fertile smell still oozes from the black peat as our feet cut into it, and the silvery granite of distant tors still shimmers in the changing light. My physical experience, however, is different.

In previous adventures, any discomfort was just a minor distraction from an exhilarating challenge. This time, pain, raw and urgent, dominates my thoughts: the pain of the moment; anticipated pain; remembered pain; pain that might never even happen. I don't know why, but it's become a neurosis. Will this jar my knees? Is nausea about to overwhelm me? Will I slip and sprain an ankle? Are my hips seizing up? Will the coming descent torture my bruised toes?

I never used to be such a wimp. Now even the wind bothers me: it slices through me, icing my bones. It's almost as if I'm a different person: a shambling skeleton, with hologram muscles where there used to be real ones. The only part of me that still seems solid is my midriff, marginally thicker than it used to be but currently feeling like a vast, cumbersome load.

At one point, as we battle our way down a thickly tangled wooded slope, I think I hear Gavin shout from ahead: 'I can see the cars.' When I realise he'd actually said: 'I can see the path' – the cars are still many miles away – I feel tempted to lie down and cry. But I dare not stop – what if they left me here? I feel frightened by my weakness, like an old lion suddenly sensing the approaching moment when it won't be able to catch its prey any more.

I've come to Devon in the hope of picking up a few tips about how to run well in later life, but I fear I'm out of my depth. Jo and Gavin coach runners in several age groups, including, these days, the middle-aged. Gavin is the main coach: qualified, full-time and highly experienced. Jo provides back-up, inspiration and mentoring – subject to the competing demands of her own training, the needs of two school-age children and a wide variety of (mostly unpaid) roles as a kind of ambassador for running. Between them, they should have lots to teach me. Yet it's hard to see what advice they can give today beyond 'Go away and come back when you're in better shape.'

In the circumstances, they are as tactful as it's possible to be. 'Don't put everything down to age-related changes,' Jo advises gently. 'Sometimes you think: I'm getting older, I can't run. But if you think, "Right, what training have I been doing in the last three months?" Maybe you haven't really done much. So don't you think that if you were young you'd be running badly as well?'

It's particularly easy, she says, to take speed for granted. 'I remember coming back to the track when I was in my twenties, and for some reason I'd done nothing but jog all winter, and when I tried running 200m it was taking me about forty seconds. So don't just think of yourself as old. Think to yourself, "Even if I was a young athlete, I'd be running slow if I wasn't bothering to do any speed work." Even in your twenties you're going to get slower if you just go for a nice jog all the time.'

Even so, she concedes, mere age does tend to make things harder; again, she focuses on her own weakness, not mine. 'My muscle strength isn't as good as it was. I seem to get less power off each stride, less rebound from each footstep. It's weird: when I'm actually doing it, it feels the same. I feel like I'm putting in the same exertion. It's just the clock that's changed at the end.'

Some of this is attributable to physiological deterioration. Some isn't. Life changes too, as the years go by. 'I have different priorities as I get older,' says Jo. 'Obviously I'm not going to make the Olympics any more, so if there's stuff going on with the kids, that's going to be my priority. Once I would have juggled things around, but it gets a bit irrational to say I'm not going to the beach because I've got to do my track session.'

It's the same for most of us. We lose our appetite for really focused training, not because we're lazy or feeble but because we have other things to do. In due course we reap the physiological consequences – which often means finding that we actually have become lazy and feeble.

Jo's advice is that, to rekindle my hunger, I should set myself a goal, ambitious but realistic. For example, she says: 'I'm never going to get a PB, but I would like to run faster this year than I did last year.' When you're getting older, that's harder than it sounds. The default option, if you don't ease off, is to get slightly slower. Actual net improvement requires serious, sustained, targeted training. But Jo is also realistic, suggesting that, in my case, it might not be wise to plunge straight away into a full-scale programme of intense speed training. Instead, she advises, I should begin by simply re-familiarising myself with what it feels like to run fast. 'It doesn't have to be a big deal. For example, I recently went up to a flat bit in the forest and thought, "I'm going to do my intervals here." It wasn't very precise, and I'm not putting any pressure on how quick I'm doing them. I just did ten times two minutes, back and forth, feeling my way into it. It feels really nice, because you're ticking off two minutes at a time. And by doing that you get the feeling of having used your legs through a larger range of motion, because you just naturally open your stride length.'

All this sounds very sensible, and is expressed in terms that – in contrast to much training advice – I can easily relate to. But training for improvement can wait for another day. Right now, my only goal is survival.

Yet one tip does make an immediate difference. 'The important thing', says Jo, 'is to keep going out there and enjoying yourself.' This sounds absurd. The important thing, surely, is to stop? Yet she's right: my negative fixation on the morning's discomforts verges on complacency, or perhaps even idiocy. Running is a privilege, especially if you're still able to do it in middle age and beyond, and access to wild, beautiful places is another great good fortune. And part of Jo's secret, I realise, is that she doesn't take the good things in her life for granted. Family, friends, community, running, the Devon landscape: she remains grateful for them all; and, as a result, still approaches life with a visible spring in her step. 'It's so nice just to be out in the natural environment,' she enthuses, and I realise that this is the running lesson I most urgently need right now. My self-pity is slowing me down.

So I make a conscious effort to focus outwards. I let myself be mesmerised by the complexity of the crisp-textured lichen on the boulders; savour the springy, forgiving texture of the ground underfoot; enjoy the warmth that still leaks from the heather's stringy remains; and marvel at the crazy lurchings of wind-tossed birds, gusted and scattered in the cold sky. I notice, too, the carefree body language of Jo's running: heels flying behind her, ponytail bouncing wildly. Where my movements are pinched and timid, she runs eagerly, fearlessly, with the happy abandon of a child. That's what I should be doing – if I could.

Defeatist thoughts still flicker on the edge of my consciousness, like notifications on my phone. Pain. Nausea. Cold. A widening gap in front of me. Each jab of awareness reminds me of my weakness. So I force myself to ignore them; and, gradually, I notice that I am thinking a little less about not being able to get enough air into my lungs and a little more about what that air tastes like. It's hard to feel wholly miserable when you're trying to identify flavours in a clean Dartmoor breeze: wind-dried turf, damp moss, warm lichen.

And then, unexpectedly, I feel a stab of positivity. Maybe I'm not doing that badly, all things considered. After all, I reason, I am not just a mediocre runner. I am a mediocre runner who is carrying an invisible load. It's not my only problem, or the biggest. But that unseen burden of age explains much of my new-found frailty;

and it's not my fault. Of course I'm slow and suffering: what I'm trying to do is difficult.

This thought gives me a kind of strength. The fact that I've been finding this morning's run a stomach-churning, joint-torturing struggle doesn't invalidate my efforts, I remind myself. It just gives them context. Just as fell-runners are up against the invisible obstacle of gravity, or ultra-runners up against the obstacle of the enormous distances they have already run (unnoticed by onlookers who mistake them for unusually slow joggers), so the runner who carries an invisible load of age is up against a brutal physical reality.

Fell-runners and ultra-runners aren't lesser versions of 'proper' runners. They're just a particular kind of runner, striving for excellence in a slightly different version of the sport. Shouldn't we think of old runners in the same way?

Sporting achievement is not diminished by arbitrary obstacles. They are the essence of sporting competition. 'Think how much easier it would be if the goal was bigger in football or the net was lower in tennis,' Noora Ronkainen once told me. 'But the obstacles are the point. Even in the 400 metres, you start and finish in the same place. You could just sit on the grass . . .'

She is right. It's meant to be difficult. Was Ed Moses a less legendary athlete than Michael Johnson, because his 400m world records involved hurdles and, as a result, were several seconds slower than Johnson's at the same distance? Of course not. The greatness lies in the degree to which each man approached the absolute limits of physical possibility.

It's the same with ageing. It's not a reason for defeatism;

nor is it something to be embarrassed about. It's just one more arbitrary sporting constraint. Why should it be the only such constraint that makes the contest less credible? And in that case, why beat myself up about falling behind? Sod it. I'm doing my best, and I'm proud of it.

Gavin interrupts my musings with some well-intended but unwelcome news: 'Sorry, but I'm just going to add on a bit extra to the loop, so you can enjoy the view from up there.' It's not the first time he's made such a suggestion, and I haven't always been as grateful as I should. This time, however, why not? I'm done with feeling sorry for myself.

OK, great, I say cheerfully. I know that my running will become more pathetic with each extra mile. It will become more pathetic with each extra year, too, if I remain a runner. But why should I feel ashamed of either? Just as long as I don't give up.

Eventually we reach a particularly exposed tor, where the wind almost blows us from the high granite slabs. Then we head off down what I think (mistakenly) is the final steep descent. The wind is biting into us from straight ahead now, the coldest it's been all morning. But I'm feeling too defiant to be feeble. Cold? It's just one more invisible enemy: bring it on. I didn't ask for these extra burdens. I'm just carrying them, and, as it happens, finding it tough. But that's because they are tough. And yet, even so, I'm still going. And, as I force my aching joints into a semblance of a light-footed run, that feels like a kind of victory.

The slope grows steeper still, yet I seem to be floating down it, rather gently. The icy wind lashes our faces, but it no longer seems to cut through me. Instead, I realise, it is bearing me up, invisibly.

When we reach the bottom, it turns out that this isn't quite the end. I should have guessed. The car park I spotted from higher up isn't the one I've been longing for, and there are several miles of foot-tangling hillside forest 'path' still to be negotiated. But I'm a lot less disappointed than I would have been half-an-hour ago; in fact, I'm enjoying myself. The slower pace suits me, and this changed environment is irresistibly absorbing: the stillness of the narrow valley; the dry, crumbling, knee-deep leaves, strangely noiseless; and the river Dart below us, vigorous, leaping and overflowing. The stabbing pains in my joints have resolved themselves into a generalised numbness, and there's time to chat: about running, life, parenthood, ageing and much else besides.

I know that we will stop eventually, just as I know that, eventually, my days of running will come to an end. I should make the most of both while I can.

Near the end, Jo says: 'You're a good runner. You can happily keep going.' Both statements are palpably untrue, but they have a ridiculously powerful effect. Happiness and self-belief flood through me, and when we do finally reach the right car park, I almost feel as though I have won something.

I haven't of course. I have merely survived. But even that is a start. They send me away with a headful of wise, digestible advice and, more importantly, a heartful of hope. If I stick to the former – who knows? – maybe even I could be better next year; and if I maintain the latter, perhaps that will motivate me to do so. Both are big 'ifs'; but, in the meantime, the morning has given me one other reward: I am feeling a long-forgotten sense of runner's self-respect. This might seem odd, given my abject performance, but I cling to it as if it were a hard-won medal, and there is nothing fragile about it. I have understood where I stand. I am slower because I am older, because I am carrying an invisible load. If I carry it bravely and defiantly, that will be a cause for pride, not embarrassment.

A whole new world of running possibility seems to open up.

9

Giants

The Milton Evergreen Cemetery, in a prosperous sub-
urb of Toronto, is a lush, park-like space, with
avenues of leafy maple trees and acres of neatly mown
grass. Nearly 9,000 Canadians have been buried there
over the past 140 years, but the low, granite headstones
are mostly so sober in design, so neatly distributed
around its plentiful space, that you barely notice them.
Instead, you see the trees, and the benches, and the dec-
orative wood carvings; and the flat, straight, asphalt
paths, on which even the unsteadiest of mourners can
safely take a contemplative stroll. When they do, the
chances are they'll be following in the footsteps of a man
who was arguably the greatest old runner of all.

Ed Whitlock, who in 2017 was laid to rest in a modest
grave in the south-west corner, spent much of his later
life training on these quiet paths. Every day he would be
there, a small old man with floppy white hair and a stooping gait, usually in the same threadbare kit and the same
ancient pair of Brooks trainers, endlessly repeating the
same circuit of around a third of a mile. He didn't measure it precisely; nor did he time himself or even count
the laps. He just jogged round and round it, possibly no

faster than at 10-minute mile pace, practising 'running for a long time' for up to three hours a day.

It wasn't a full circuit of the cemetery, because he left out a section with a slope in it. He didn't like hills. So his asphalt route was flat as well as smooth, and he tended to stare at it as he ran. Asked what was going through his head, he answered, in deadpan tones that were as English as his politely shambolic manner, that he was usually thinking, 'When will this be over?' or, 'Why is this taking so long?' Asked why he didn't find somewhere more interesting to run, he replied: 'That would require a degree of organisation that I don't possess.' Yet by the time he took up occupancy of his 4ft by 9ft plot – its gravestone surmounted by a cast of his old trainers – he had become the most famous Masters athlete in the world.

Born in 1931, Whitlock grew up in Kingston upon Thames. He was a decent junior cross-country runner – he once beat the great Gordon Pirie – but was plagued by Achilles tendon problems and gave up running soon after graduating as a mining engineer in 1952. He moved to Canada; married; had children; kept relatively fit and active through cycling, walking and football refereeing, and made his first tentative attempts at a running comeback in 1972, aged forty-one. He found he still had a talent for middle distances, and when the first World Masters Athletics championships was held in Toronto, he couldn't resist getting involved. It was the first of three world championships in which he competed between 1975 and 1979, winning, altogether, a silver and a gold for 1500m and a bronze at 800m.

But his right Achilles still troubled him, so he drifted into what he called 'plodding'. He ran his first marathon in 1975, aged forty-four, to support his fourteen-year-old son, Clive. They ran and finished together, amid Montreal snowdrifts, in 3:09. A few weeks later they ran another marathon, eleven minutes faster. Whitlock was hooked – especially when his younger son, Neil, caught the bug as well. In 1978 the forty-seven-year-old father ran a 2:48 marathon alongside his son, and within a year Ed had gone 17 minutes faster. But he was still only warming up.

A few years later, the Whitlocks settled in Milton. Ed continued to run to a high standard, especially after retiring from work in his early sixties and finding time to do a whole lot more training. There were plenty of scenic trails on which to do this: Milton is on the edge of the Niagara Escarpment. But after a few years Whitlock developed a preference for the local cemetery, where he could escape such hazards as traffic, dogs, snowdrifts, ice, biting winds, and the temptation to impress passers-by. A single weaving loop took him well under five minutes, so he just kept repeating it, sometimes for hours at a time. The monotony didn't bother him. Thanks to retirement – the older runner's big competitive advantage – he had all the time he needed.

Even so, he never got round to expanding his training to include practices such as stretching, speed work or weights. Generally, his approach seemed as casual as his fixed routine of daily plodding was obsessive. Each item of running kit was made to last for decades. As for diet, he ate 'whatever they're serving'. He accepted that a more scientific approach might be beneficial. But, he said, he wasn't 'sufficiently organised or ambitious' to do anything about it.

Instead, he stuck determinedly to his relentless cemetery regime, and developed a base of stamina that
empowered him to take late-life distance running to a
previously unimagined level. Over two decades from
1996, he set more than twenty world records (it's hard to
be exact, because he didn't keep track), in age groups from
M65 to M85 and at distances from 1500m to marathon,
many of which remain unbroken. But there was one particular cluster of records that made him world-famous.

The thought occurred to him as he approached his
seventieth birthday: what if he could become the first
person over seventy to run a marathon in under three
hours? This was, he insisted with his usual self-mockery,
a 'silly objective'; yet the neatness of it fascinated him. It
was, he said, 'the poor man's four-minute mile', a one-
time-only prize that was 'just sitting there waiting for
someone'. He had run a 2:51:02 marathon at sixty-eight
and a 2:52:50 at sixty-nine, so he felt that it must be within
reach. But with marathons, as anyone who has tried one
knows, everything needs to go right. Initially, it didn't.
For his first attempt, at seventy, he had a bad day and
missed out by twenty-three seconds. Then he hurt his
knee and couldn't run for a year. But finally, aged seventy-
two, he broke the barrier, with 2:59:09; and it turned out
that, even then, he was just getting into his stride.

The following year, 2004, the seventy-three-year-old
Whitlock ran 2:54:48, which the *New York Times* suggested might be the greatest marathon ever run, once
'age-grading' had been applied. Had he run that time in
the first marathon of the modern Olympics, in 1896, he
would have beaten the winner by four minutes. As

recently as 2012 you could have run 2:54:48 in the men's Olympic marathon and not come last.

In 2005, he broke three hours again, this time in 2:58:40. He was seventy-four by then. This remains the oldest age at which anyone has run a sub-three-hour marathon. Most runners, remember, can't get below three hours even in their prime.

Then, after turning seventy-five, Whitlock found a fresh bounce in his step. In one magical week in July 2006 he set four M75 world records, for the mile, 3,000m, 5,000m and 10,000m, all of which still stand. He ran some spectacularly fast marathons, notably 3:04:54 in Rotterdam as a seventy-six-year-old. Then, in 2011, he returned to Rotterdam to run 3:25:43 as an eighty-year-old, a record that he lowered to 3:15:54 in Toronto later that year. His resulting celebrity was boosted by a new clutch of world records (also still standing) at 3,000m, 5,000m and 10,000m. The attention left him 'somewhat embarrassed', he said, and he cautioned people against treating him as a role model: 'I'm not sure what I'm doing is good for me, let alone anyone else.'

Finally, in October 2016, Whitlock became the first eighty-five-year-old to break four hours for a marathon. (Most male finishers in the London Marathon, irrespective of age, are slower than that.) Once again Whitlock was at the Toronto Waterfront Marathon, this time sporting the race number '85' on his thirty-year-old vest. His barely cushioned Brooks trainers were, by contrast, a mere fifteen years old. He pronounced himself disappointed with his time of 3:56:38, which slashed thirty-eight minutes off the previous record. He had hoped to run

3:50, but 'things fell apart in the second half of the race' and he had considered quitting. And although he had hung on to achieve what no eighty-five-year-old had come close to achieving before, he felt bothered by the steepness of his recent decline: 'Only twelve years ago I was running an hour faster.'

An increasingly arthritic knee hadn't helped, but Whitlock was right to sense a wider deterioration. His performances were declining more quickly than before, although it may not have been age alone that was to blame. Perhaps, too, he had begun to feel the effects of the prostate cancer that would kill him five months later, a week after his eighty-sixth birthday.

The shock of his passing was felt far beyond Toronto. He had become an international Masters icon by then, partly on account of his apparent indestructibility. To see him brought low by death without having reached the furthest extremes of old age felt unnatural as well as sad.

The consensus was that the athletic world would not see his like again. Yet although he was certainly a one-off in his manner (Roger Robinson called him 'the most modest, droll, amiable and intelligent of all miraculous legends'), he wasn't quite the unique physiological phenomenon that some imagined. Even in Canada – even in his little corner of Canada – there were other extraordinary pensioners exploring previously unimagined limits of what it is possible for an old person to achieve as an athlete.

One of them was Keijo Taivassalo, a Finnish-born marathon runner living in Toronto. Eight years younger than Whitlock, he was less sensational in his talents but still deeply impressive. A future age-group winner of the

Boston Marathon (in 3:52:22 as an eighty-year-old in 2019) and world champion half-marathon runner (in 2:07:45 as an eighty-three-year-old in 2022), he was good enough as a seventy-year-old to compete in the marathon at the 2009 World Masters Athletics championships in Lahti, Finland – an adventure on which his daughter Tanja accompanied him.

Keijo came back without a medal, but Tanja, an exercise physiology professor then working at McGill University in Montreal, came back with an idea. She had been so impressed with what she saw that, with her colleague and future husband Russ Hepple, she co-organised a landmark study into the physiology of very old, very good athletes.

The McGill Masters study, as it is loosely known (actually it was several studies, and its data is still being analysed today), was notable in part for its extreme elitism. In its most important formulation, only fourteen athletes were studied, seven male and seven female, alongside fifteen non-athlete controls. The athletes, with an average age just under eighty, were all in the top four in the world in their events, and seven were world record-holders. Among them were Whitlock and his friend Earl Fee, a middle-distance runner and hurdler of whom we'll be hearing more shortly.

But the star of the show was Olga Kotelko, a nonagenarian ex-teacher of Ukrainian descent, from Saskatchewan in central Canada. She had won more than 700 gold medals since taking up athletics at seventy-seven and in the W90 category alone would eventually set twenty-six world records. She had also come close to scuppering the whole study, after the McGill ethics board objected to such an elderly woman taking part in such physically demanding research – but Taivassalo had eventually won them round. Kotelko had been the big sensation of the Lahti Games, winning W90 gold medals in eleven events over eight days, and setting eight world records, in disciplines including 100m (in 25.05 seconds), 200m (56.46), high jump (0.82m), long jump (1.77m), shot put (4.86m), discus (13.92m), hammer (12.91m) and javelin (13.54m), and Taivassalo's original idea had been to investigate her alone.

Kotelko, a small, modest, solidly built lady whose capable manner and reassuring smile suggested the teacher she used to be, was soon the star of the research laboratory, where she was measured for everything from VO_2 max and cardiac output to flexibility, maximal muscle strength and brain density, as well as having samples of blood and thigh muscle removed for analysis. A crowd of young students watched open-mouthed as the ninety-one-year-old bench-pressed 60lb (27.2kg). As for her laboratory results, they were as remarkable as the researchers had hoped.

Some of the numbers, such as her VO_2 max (15.5ml per kilogram of body weight per minute) and maximal heart rate (135 bpm), were hard to contextualise. There simply wasn't enough data on what was 'normal' for a ninety-one-year-old woman running on a treadmill. But there was clearly nothing remotely normal about Kotelko's muscle fibres: in her biopsy, there was no detectable evidence of mitochondrial decay at all. This was extraordinary: mitochondrial decay is considered universal in the over-sixty-fives. Yet Kotelko appeared to have some kind of resistance to it. So, to a slightly lesser extent, did other athletes in the study; both Fee and Whitlock, for example, had roughly twice as many mitochondria in their muscle cells as the non-athlete controls. The athletes weren't all in perfect health: Whitlock's blood pressure was a bit high, and Fee had suffered since his sixties from occasional tachycardia (spells of very rapid heartbeat). Compared with healthy non-athletes, however, they had significantly higher quantities of functioning motor units (which deliver nerve signals to muscles), better preservation of neuromuscular transmission stability and, as a result, better preservation of excitable muscle mass. In other words, their muscles had wasted away much less than expected and, to a surprising extent, still worked as a younger person's might.

Media coverage at the time had suggested that the study would in due course 'unlock the secrets of ageing'. It didn't, obviously. It didn't even really clarify the extent to which the subjects' remarkable physiological qualities were the cause or the effect of their sporting activities; or the extent to which their athletic gifts were genetic or acquired. It would be hard to do either without somehow finding a huge sample of octogenarians with similarly spectacular athletic potential, realised and unrealised, who could be measured against one another in relation to different variables. As for the most intriguing question of all – were the subjects' achievements attributable to athletic talent (inherited or acquired) or to some form of age-resistance (inherited or acquired)? – that, too, remained mostly unresolved.

None the less, the study turned out to be something of a watershed. A decade or so earlier, the physiology of very old athletes had been an almost laughably obscure specialism. Since the McGill study, however, it has increasingly been recognised as an important and exciting frontier of scientific inquiry. Young sciences often are, once they catch on. As Roger Robinson pointed out at the time, every time Ed Whitlock raced, he laid down 'a completely new body of potential evidence about the human ageing process'. In other words, no one had really looked at this stuff before. So there were vast areas of ignorance to be charted, with potential implications far beyond sport, and, as a result, there was and is great scope for bright and ambitious researchers to find a niche and make a name for themselves. No one sneers at old-age sport physiology today.

But the study was also a landmark for another reason: because of the sheer headline-making stature of its subjects. 'These folks really were the cream of the crop,' says Hepple, who is now professor of Physical Therapy and Muscle Biology at the University of Florida (where Taivassalo is an associate professor). Whitlock, Kotelko and Fee alone set around 120 world records between them, with performances so wildly at odds with prevailing stereotypes of 'normal' ageing that the wider world could hardly help noticing. Throw in a few of the other stars in the study – the Kansas sprinter Bob Lida; the Atlanta-based middle-distance runner Jeanne Daprano; the Vancouver marathon runner Betty Jean McHugh – and you have a truly extraordinary Golden Generation of north American late-life athletes. In marketing terms, these were the first Masters to achieve anything approaching 'crossover'.

They were not, however, the last. You don't have to be a hard-core Masters enthusiast to have heard of Gene Dykes, the seventy-three-year-old self-styled 'ultra-geezer' from Philadelphia who, in addition to being a jaw-droppingly prolific and occasionally record-breaking ultra-runner, ran four sub-three-hour marathons within twelve-and-a-half months of turning seventy in April 2018, including one, in Jacksonville, Florida, which was 25 seconds faster than Whitlock's M70 best. This was never ratified as a world record because the race, unlike the course, turned out not to have the proper paperwork from USA Track & Field. But no one seriously doubted that this was septuagenarian distance-running at a level reached previously only by Whitlock – any more than they did when, in May 2022, a seventy-one-year-old Dutchman called Jo Schoonbroodt ran the Maasmarathon of Visé, in Liège, Belgium, in 2:54:19, which if ratified will be the new world record.

Schoonbroodt, who started jogging to get his cholesterol levels down when he was thirty-six and didn't start chasing records until decades later, attributes his success to the fact that 'Everything is new to me'; and to the fact that most of his training is done slowly, for pleasure, on trails; and, modestly, to his use in races of carbon-plated Asics shoes that Whitlock could never have imagined. As for Dykes, his guiding philosophy is simply to 'do a little bit more each year – whether it's further, or faster, or more adventurous.' Speaking to me during a rare break from training and racing (he had just broken a shoulder blade after tripping in a trail race), Dykes, a retired computer programmer with a geeky grin, enthused cheerfully and tirelessly about the pleasure he gets from his still relatively new hobby, which he took up in his mid-fifties. But the idea that spurs him on, he explained, is a simple urge to improve. 'The most healthy competition you can have is to beat that guy in the mirror,' he said. 'Whatever he did the year before, you've got to top it in the next one.' Many runners will recognise the motivating power of this kind of approach – when we start out. For most of us, however, it stops working long before our seventies. Dykes – who also holds records for 50km, 100 miles and twenty-four-hours and for being the oldest person ever to complete all three major US 200-milers in the same year – shows that it doesn't have to.

Nor is it just at the long-distance end of the spectrum that stirring late-life goals and achievements are possible, as another Masters giant, Charles Allie, proves. If the name means nothing to you, remember it now: this is one of the most impressive runners on the planet, as an athlete and as a person. A retired industrial art shop teacher from Pitts-burgh, Allie has twice been voted World Masters Male Athlete of the Year, in 2013 and 2018, and you wouldn't bet against his winning the title for a third time once the Masters circuit is properly up and running again. He was a few months short of seventy-five when I spoke to him, and, as Masters athletes tend to do, he was looking forward to joining a new age group (although his birthday would come just too late for the 2022 world championships). He explained that he 'started slowly' in Masters athletics, when he was forty. Over the past couple of decades, however, he had won multiple world titles at 100m, 200m and 400m, notably in the M65 and M70 categories. He had also set numerous world records, especially at his favourite distance, the 400m. His big dream, however, was an even greater pinnacle: to hold simultaneous M75 world records in all three sprint distances – itself an unprecedented achievement – including, he hoped, the world's first sub-60-second 400m by a seventy-five-year-old.

In a book littered with world records, such words may

evoke less wonder than they ought to. So it is worth pausing to consider what such an achievement would mean. The absolute world record for the one-lap event, set by Wayde van Niekerk in 2016, is 43.03 seconds, but only the absolute cream of the elite (i.e. six of the last thirty-two Olympic finalists) can break 44 seconds. The British record is 44.35; the British junior record is 45.36. Generally, you have to be a seriously gifted and committed sprinter to get under fifty seconds – and at several recent Olympics there has been a competitor or two in the heats who has failed to do even that. There are also plenty of keen and talented runners out there who couldn't even break one minute for one lap, ever, at any age.

Yet Allie, in May 2013, at a South-Eastern Masters meet in Raleigh, North Carolina, ran 400m in 56.09 – as a sixty-five-year-old. This was barely 8 seconds slower than Allie's lifetime best as a college athlete more than forty years earlier, and nearly 2 seconds faster than the M65 world record set in 1995 by the great Earl Fee. It was also an astonishing 9 seconds less than Allie's age in years. (To put that remarkable detail in context: running 400m in 'less than your age' is one of the great fitness challenges for men over fifty. Only an exceptionally fast, exceptionally well-preserved athlete could even contemplate it – while for women, and men under fifty, it appears to be physio logically impossible. Yet Allie just blasted his age by 9 clear seconds.)

Five-and-a-half years later, as a seventy-one-year-old, Allie ran the same distance in 57.26, at the world championships in Málaga, Spain. This was more than 2 seconds faster than the previous M70 world record, and, this time, nearly 14 seconds faster than his age. You wouldn't think it from talking to him – he's modest, approachable and self-deprecating – but these are performances so far ahead of the curve that they may never even have been imagined before. And yet the best might be yet to come. He's still in peak condition, still capable of doing a lap of the track in under a minute, and when I spoke to him he appeared to have every chance of achieving his objectives in the new age group. It's a huge challenge, and there's an awful lot that can go wrong when you're seventy-five (whereas for the 100m, in particular, he really needs everything to go right). But if he does achieve that elusive world record treble – including a sub-60-second 400m – he'll have a good claim to be ranked among the very greatest athletes ever, of any age.

Allie wasn't in the McGill study, but he was extensively examined at around the same time in a study at the University of Pittsburgh, as part of an ongoing project called the Performance and Research Initiative for Masters Athletes. 'They put me through this whole week-long process,' Allie told me in 2021. 'I was on the treadmill for a whole half-hour,' he laughed. (He laughs a lot.) 'They took blood, gave me a full body scan, did bone density tests, took my blood pressure – everything you could think of. It was like a free medical.'

Predictably, he was found to be in absurdly good condition, the most striking points of his data being an exceptionally high proportion of fast-twitch muscle fibres (73.7 per cent), and a very fast metabolism. 'I burn more in my metabolism when I'm at rest than most people do when they're actually participating in something.'

As for Gene Dykes, he too was studied in exhaustive physiological detail, following his unratified marathon

world best at Jacksonville in 2018. In his case, the researchers were based at the University of Delaware in Newark,
New Jersey. Their findings, published in the *New England
Journal of Medicine* in April 2019, were controversial. No
one disputed the data demonstrating Dykes's superb cardiovascular and metabolic health, or the fact that his VO_2
max (46.9ml per kilogram of body weight per minute)
was insanely high for his age. (The average for an age-
matched male would be about 26ml per kg per minute.)
But even 46.9 didn't seem high enough for a man who
could run a 2:54:23 marathon. The team hypothesised that
Dykes's secret was an ability to sustain an exceptionally
high percentage of maximum output – 93 per cent rather
than the 80 to 85 per cent typically seen in elite marathon
runners – throughout the race. This provoked corres-
pondence from other scientists who felt that this was
physiologically impossible. Research elsewhere suggested
that the original researchers were probably right, but we
will get to that in the next chapter.

Meanwhile, there are plenty of other physiological rid-
dles to ponder. It seems pretty clear, for example, that
most of the all-time greats of old-age running are bene-
fiting in some way from what might be called 'slow
ageing'. You can see this at a cellular level in, for example,
those barely decayed muscle fibres. You can also see it in
the way these athletes' relative performances improve as
their careers progress. Charles Allie was 'good but not
great' as a college athlete, unable to challenge Olympic-
bound contemporaries such as Bob Hayes, Lee Evans,
Tommy Smith and John Carlos. As the decades have
passed, however, he has begun to outstrip his rivals by an
almost indecent distance. Is the competition less intense?

Of course. That is what slow ageing means. In terms of 'functional age' (that is, what you can still do), everyone is declining; but others are declining at a much faster rate.

Earl Fee, who is still setting records today as a ninety-three-year-old, puts it succinctly. 'My main training secret', he says, 'is to age more slowly than my rivals.'

But is it really a question of training secrets – or the luck of the genetic draw? One analysis of the McGill data looked at the length of its subjects' telomeres, those protein caps on our chromosomes whose length is a marker of ageing. The elite athletes in the study all had telomeres of much the same length: not super-long, as you might expect in people who were ageing at a dramatically slower rate than their peers, but slightly longer than average – just like the Super Seniors in Angela Brooks-Wilson's Healthy Ageing Study (mentioned in Chapter 4). This wasn't surprising. All of them *were* 'super seniors', in the sense of having dodged major diseases. Given the amount of training the athletes were doing, however, it was hard not to ask a more speculative question: were the McGill athletes born with just-right telomeres? Or had their intensive training somehow manipulated them into their 'Goldilocks' length?

Mark Tarnopolsky, the adventure-racing Canadian professor quoted in Chapter 4, has been looking into this area for years. 'At the end of the day', he says, 'maintaining the length of the telomeres comes down to optimal mitochondrial health.' Mitochondria, often nicknamed 'the powerhouse of the cell', are the cellular sub-units that convert food into energy. They accumulate damage as we age, and physical functionality declines as this happens; but they thrive on athletic training. 'Mitochondria are a key player,' says Tarnopolsky. 'There's clearly a link between mitochondrial dysfunction and many of the essential components of human ageing, including the muscles' ability to extract oxygen from the blood. There's also senescence activation, there's oxidative stress activation, there's inflammation activation. And there's telomere shortening. So maintaining healthy mitochondria, and stimulating the production of telomerase, is crucial. And you can stimulate that through exercise.'

Taivassalo and Hepple have also focused on mitochondria in much of their subsequent work, often using new analytical techniques to 'dive down deeper' into data gathered from the McGill superstars. One recent paper concluded that 'mitochondrial pathways are key to maintaining a high level of physical function in advanced age.' They noted, however, that some of the 176 proteins related to mitochondria that were 'differentially expressed' in high-functioning Masters athletes were not known to be responsive to exercise. This implied that 'the mechanisms responsible for their high function remain unclear.' Perhaps, they speculated, the athletes actually owed their enviable physical state not just to their training but to 'a fortuitous combination of genetics and environmental factors beyond exercise'.

'My sense is that these folk really are unique,' says Hepple. 'There's some unique ageing biology in there, and we don't really know what it is.' There are, he admits, some in the scientific community who disapprove of research with so many unknowns and unknowables. 'People sometimes look at what we're doing and say, "Well, it's a fishing expedition." But it's a fishing expedition being done with humans who are living better than most of us could ever hope to. So to me it's worthwhile, because we just might catch a good fish.'

For most of us, meanwhile, for practical purposes, the answers may not matter very much. We can take it as read that, like all sporting world-beaters, the giants of Masters running started off with some huge natural advantages. Otherwise, we would all be champions. We can also take it as read that smart lifestyle choices, including training regimes, have contributed to their late-life well-being and athleticism. Otherwise, why would any older athletes bother to train? And while there is not a lot we can do about it if we don't share the world-beaters' genetic good fortune, it is both reasonable and prudent to look at their examples for insights about training and lifestyle that might help us to slow our own decline.

But this isn't easy either, because we face the same problem as the scientists: there are simply too few people achieving this degree of age-proofing for our observations of cause and effect to have much statistical reliability. Sometimes we think we discern patterns. More often than not, we are spotting coincidences, and what seem like common threads end up leading nowhere.

For example: Fee and Kotelko were both born close to the remote Saskatchewan prairie town of Elstow; Fee and Whitlock both spent much of their lives in Toronto suburbs (Fee's, Mississauga, is just a dozen miles from Milton); Whitlock and Kotelko both came from relatively long-lived families (Whitlock's Uncle Arthur was Britain's oldest man). But that's as far as it went. None of these statements applied universally.

Similarly: quite a few of the late-life superstars mentioned above seem to have drawn strength from long, happy marriages (Whitlock, Dykes, Allie), yet others (Kotelko, Fee) have had the opposite experience. Several have been motivated by strong religious faith; others never mention it. Some knew physical hardship as children (Kotelko, Fee, Allie), yet others, such as Whitlock, grew up in relative comfort.

Fee and Whitlock present a particularly intriguing pattern of parallels and contrasts. Fee, who was eighty-one at the time of the McGill study, was a retired nuclear engineer; Whitlock was a retired mining engineer. Just like Whitlock, Fee showed promise as young runner, took several decades off (but stayed reasonably fit); returned to running in middle age (fifty-seven in his case) when his two sons, like Whitlock's, showed an interest in the sport; and went on, like Whitlock, to accumulate an improbably large collection of records and titles.

Yet when we get to the heart of the matter – lifestyle and training – the parallels vanish. Fee's approach, it turns out, is the exact opposite to Whitlock's. He believes in very short, very intense training sessions – rarely more than twenty minutes at a time. He calculates everything, keeping a detailed training log and planning each new record like a military campaign. He takes thirteen different vitamin supplements a day, avoids sugar, starch and processed foods, and sticks meticulously to his day-by-day weekly diet plan: for example, porridge made with steel-cut oats with walnuts and pumpkin seeds for breakfast four days a week, but eggs with baked red potato and beans three days a week, washed down with two-and-a-half glasses of water with flaxseed. He believes, broadly speaking, that the ageing body struggles to tolerate a high volume of training, but can still manage high intensity. So he would typically do three track sessions per week, based on a series of short, intense sprints with longish recovery intervals, and on non-running days would just keep things ticking over with low-impact activities such as walking, swimming or aquacise (i.e. running or walking in the water). He is an enthusiastic stretcher, doing his first stretching exercises of the day before getting out of bed, and also makes extensive use of a foam roller to massage stiff or sore muscles. As a result, he says, he has largely been spared the shortening of the stride that afflicts most older runners. He also does lots of strength exercises – press-ups, sit-ups, rubber-band resistance exercises for the legs – but since turning ninety he has more or less given up actual weights, which leave his legs too tired for the next day.

If you want to know more, Fee, who is already plotting which records he will target when he becomes an M95 in March 2024, has written several books about his running, notably the exhaustive *The Complete Guide to Running: How to Be a Champion from 9 to 90* (420 pages) and the encyclopaedic *100 Years Young the Natural Way* (664 pages). I know several successful athletes who swear by his teachings, and others who find them unreadable. What's beyond dispute is that his leave-nothing-to-chance philosophy works for him. He has twice been voted World Masters Athlete of the Year, in 2005 and 2019, and the last time I looked he had sixty world records to his name, mostly in tough events such as 400m, 800m, 1500m and long hurdles. He also has the distinction of being the oldest man to run 400m in less than his age: 89.15 seconds as a ninety-year-old in 2020.

Yet it is also hard to dispute that Fee's approach to

keeping old age at bay, through high intensity training and obsessively healthy living, has almost nothing in common with Whitlock's.

The McGill study suggested that there were benefits to both approaches. Fee had preserved more fast-twitch muscle fibres, as you might expect from someone whose best distances are between 400m and a mile. Whitlock had the most spectacular VO_2 max: 54. Perhaps each had the best approach for his range of distances, but if you spread the net slightly wider that pattern blurs too. Gene Dykes, the current miraculous old man of marathon-running, has a happy-go-lucky approach much like Whitlock's. His training regime is based largely on vast mileage – he races most weekends, often in major ultras, and aims to cover up to 1,500 miles a year in races alone. He boasts of an anything-goes approach to nutrition ('Junk food shivers in its shoes when it sees me coming') and has a comprehensive set of training no-go zones: 'No stretching, no flexibility, no weights, no core work, no cross-training.' He does employ a trainer, John Goldthorp, but this appears to be mainly for motivational purposes: 'I couldn't think of letting him down.' His technical secret is to 'get out and run'.

Jo Schoonbroodt takes a similarly casual approach: 'You have to start with a feeling of freedom, and not with a feeling of "I must do this, I must do that." You have to enjoy your training.' Yet other long-distance Masters superstars incline more towards Fee than towards Whitlock. When Mariko Yugeta became the first woman over sixty to run a sub-three-hour marathon (improved in January 2021 to 2:52:13 as a sixty-two-year-old), she specifically attributed her late-life success to becoming as meticulous in her planning as the professionals. 'When you're going for a world record,' Japan's newest running sensation told the Tokyo-based US journalist Brett Larner, 'you have to read up on what other top people are doing and look for what you can apply to your own running.' In her case this meant adapting not just her training (more miles, more hills) but also her nutrition (more liver, more maguro, more red meat), her kit (state-of-the-art Nike Vaporflys) and her recovery (now including acupuncture, massage and hot springs).

Earl Fee would approve, but the seeker of common threads is left with an unhelpful tangle. Different approaches suit different runners. It's the same with the seemingly obvious observation that many of the greatest older runners didn't start running seriously until well into middle age. Many of the giants mentioned here (e.g. Kotelko, Dykes, McHugh, Daprano) were late starters; others (Whitlock, Fee) quit in their twenties and then started afresh decades later. Dykes, who ran his first marathon at fifty-eight, considers this a crucial part of his winning formula: 'If you want to run really well when you're old,' he told me, 'don't run really hard when you're young.' There are, however, significant exceptions, including Allie, Lida, Yugeta and Guido Müller (the great German long hurdler who set world records in every five-year age group from M45 to M75), all of whom have run pretty seriously all their lives. 'The important thing,' Allie advised me, 'is to keep going.'

So much for patterns; yet the quest is not entirely futile. In three notable respects, most of the great old Masters do resemble one another. First: pretty much all of them, I think, are very active people. Even when not training, they are rarely sedentary. 'Once I get up I'm on the go,' says Allie, echoing what dozens of older athletes have told me. A neat, bald man with a trimmed grey beard and a gleaming white smile, he has been retired for years, yet he's always busy. If he's not training, or coaching the young athletes at his club, or racing Corvettes, he is using his industrial design skills. 'I'm always doing projects, for me, for other people. I'm kind of like a handyman. I sleep well at night because I'm basically exhausted.'

A second common trait in these older champions is a forward-facing attitude – by which I mean that there is no hint in them of the jadedness that lesser runners often feel as they age. No voice whispers to them that they can never match the heights they have already reached. As they see it, their finest hour is yet to come.

This may reflect – again, almost without exception – an absence of life-defining sporting achievement earlier in life. Some of them didn't do running at all when they were young, and have thus been able to enjoy the late-life motivation that comes from novelty and sustained, rapid improvement. Others did compete in their youth, but with less success than they would have liked. Whitlock's early athletic ambitions were curtailed by injury; so were Fee's. Müller missed out on Olympic qualification by half a second. Yugeta, meanwhile, had to dial down her youthful passion for marathon-running when marriage and motherhood intervened, yet never lost the sense that she was capable of something special in the sport. Watching on television as a twenty-six-year-old in 1984 when Joan Benoit Samuelson won the first women's Olympic marathon, Yugeta said to herself: 'If things had been different, maybe that could have been me.' That's a useful kind of frustration for a runner to take into later life. When your moment finally comes, you seize it.

'As one gets older, there is a feeling that time is running out,' says Fee, whose austere, methodical manner conceals a poet's heart. (He has published several volumes of poetry.) 'So each hour becomes more precious.' And with this awareness, he spends hour after hour trying to become the best athlete he can possibly be.

This brings us to the third trait that the great Masters champions share: a breathtaking capacity for hard work. The guiding principle of Bob Lida's training was that if he didn't feel by the end that he was about to throw up, he hadn't worked hard enough. Ed Whitlock sometimes ran three hours a day for weeks at a time. Gene Dykes tops up his quality-focused 50-mile-a-week training schedule with around forty hard races a year, which in 2018 included seven marathons and five ultramarathons. Jo Schoonbroodt ran 4,450 miles in 2021 (about 85 miles a week), which is 'more than double what I did in my car'; Mariko Yugeta runs up to 115 miles a week, many of them on the slopes of Mount Fuji. 'If you want to succeed,' says Fee, 'you have to work for it.'

Obviously this formula is more compelling if you know you have enough natural talent for competitive success to be a realistic goal. But success takes many forms, and seriously hard training brings rewards for also-rans too – especially in old age. 'When I travel,' says Allie, 'especially on the world level, I see guys my age, and we're all like friends, but they know they have no chance of winning, and yet they turn up regardless. And that inspires me. I never want to get to the point where I won because I was the only one in my age group.'

Most of us, whatever our age, under-estimate the extent to which we short-change ourselves by under-training.

The typical recreational runner does barely a fifth of the training mileage of an elite runner. We have good reasons for that, but it also helps explain why we're so much slower. Then, in old age, our habits and priorities change. Sometimes there's an opportunity to train a bit more, but often we never try it because we under-estimate our potential.

And that, perhaps, is the real significance of the golden generation of North Americans who inspired the McGill study, and of the latter-day giants who have followed them. They show us that our sense of what is impossible may be exaggerated. To see them as freaks is to miss the point: just as it would be missing the point to think of Roger Bannister or Emil Zátopek as freaks. They were pioneers, whose examples emboldened others to shake off the old self-limiting narratives, and hundreds have emulated their achievements. Similarly, Allie, Dykes, Fee and the others have shown the way, suggesting to the rest of us that, as Olga Kotelko used to tell people, 'You have more to give than you realise.'

But even she might have been surprised at the ambitions of some of today's giants-in-the-making.

10

Pie in the sky

Tommy Hughes is a couple of months older than me, and several light years faster. I'm pretty sure he always has been, although our paths didn't cross until we were both sixty. Unlike me, he is short, lean, muscular and shaven-headed, and – in further contrast to me – you can see at a glance that he is an athlete who takes his running seriously.

You may have heard of him. His achievements in recent years have earned him a degree of global fame. In the village he grew up in, however, he's been a celebrity for decades.

He still lives there: Maghera, or just outside it, in Northern Ireland's Catholic heartlands between Derry/Londonderry and Belfast. He is a bus driver's son, the oldest of eight children, who drifted into running after marrying young, putting on weight and struggling to make the first team of his local Gaelic football club.

He ran his first marathon in 1982, aged twenty-two. He had barely trained – just three 4-mile runs a week – yet still managed 3:01:28. He trained a bit harder and within a year improved to 2:35 – by which time running had become the best thing in his life. Life in Maghera in the 1980s was overshadowed by the Troubles – 'It was mad

here. There was shooting going on . . .' – and by reces-
sion. Tommy completed an apprenticeship as an electrician
but couldn't find permanent employment. So, stuck on
the dole, he poured his pent-up passion, energy and
brain power into running. He studied the latest training
techniques, upped his weekly mileage to 100 miles or
more, and tried to train both smart and hard. The effect
was startling and sustained. In 1984 he broke two-and-a-
half hours for the first time, winning the Derry Marathon
in 2:24; the following year he won it again, in 2:19. Then,
in 1988, he won the Belfast Marathon, the Melbourne
Marathon and, most spectacularly, the Marrakech Marathon, in a seriously fast 2:15:48. Ever since, he's been
known locally as the Marrakech Express.

He was selected for the 1992 Olympics in Barcelona,
but a stress fracture in his foot put an end to any medal
hopes. He recovered quickly enough to take part, however, and was delighted to finish in seventy-second place,
completing his final lap in the Olympic stadium with a
huge grin on his face.

That could have been the end of Tommy's running
story. He had been a more-or-less full-time athlete for
getting on for a decade; he had surprised himself and his
friends and family by becoming an Olympian; and when
he came home there was a job opportunity waiting for
him. There were friends, too, and girls, and pubs where a
handsome young man with such a friendly smile would
always be welcome. So he said goodbye to life as an elite
international athlete and rejoined the normal world –
complete with young man's indulgences such as beer,
cigarettes and late-night kebabs.

He didn't quit running entirely, however, and, lifestyle

notwithstanding, he was still fast enough to win the 1998 Belfast Marathon, at the age of thirty-eight, in 2:23:33. But his life no longer revolved around the sport. Instead, he grew into the roles of married father of four and full-time electrician, whose developing specialist skills eventually took him wherever the work was: 'all over England, Ireland, Scotland, even China and Saudi Arabia and stuff like that. I lived out of a suitcase for years.'

Then it came round to 2008, and the thought suddenly appeared in Tommy's forty-eight-year-old head that he might have one more shot at glory. 'It was the Belfast Marathon coming up, and because I'd won it in 1988 and I won it again in 1998, I thought to myself, "Wouldn't it be nice to win it again in 2008?" So I decided to come back to running.'

For a few weeks, he trained as intensely as he had trained for the Olympics, twice a day or more and, although there was no time to reach Olympic fitness, the race went pretty well. But with a pack of leading Kenyans and Ethiopians up against him the best he could manage was sixth, twelve minutes behind the winner. Even so, his time, 2:28:38, was remarkably good for a forty-eight-year-old. 'Then I thought, "In another two years I'll be fifty. I'd love to be the number one marathon runner when I'm fifty."'

It took him a while to get back to the highest level, but in 2010 he was good enough to win the Robin Hood Marathon, in Nottingham, in 2:29:12. He then benefited from a period of relative stability in his working life, from 2011 to 2014, when he spent so much time in Leicester that he joined a local running club, Leicester Coritanians. Yet time didn't stop, and gains made in training were easily eroded by the incoming tide of ageing, especially when exacerbated by too many evenings unwinding in the pub. In 2011, aged fifty-one, Tommy improved his Belfast Marathon placing to fifth, but his time had slipped to 2:33:16. The following year he improved his time to 2:29:43, but his placing had slipped to eighth.

Then, in 2013, the Derry/Londonderry Marathon was revived – now rebranded as the Walled City Marathon – and Tommy spotted a fresh goal. 'I won it in 1984 and 1985, but then it stopped, so I couldn't make it three in a row. So when they brought it back, I thought, well, I'll have another go here.' It was, he says, 'just another pie-in-the-sky thing', but having set his mind to it, he went for it. He was up against a much fancied, much younger, local runner, Greg Roberts, but after a ferocious duel over the first 14 miles or so the older man's greater mental resilience began to tell. Tommy completed his hat-trick in 2:30:32.

It was arguably his most impressive athletic achievement so far. Almost immediately afterwards, however, age caught up with him. He kept training, but 'I began to struggle with paces that I'd been doing beforehand. I'd be going: "Am I getting older faster than I thought I was?"' His energy levels plummeted, and he began to suffer from depression, exacerbated by 'real bad mood swings'. And this in turn merged, gradually, with a more dangerous problem. 'I've always struggled with alcohol, but when I was a full-time runner I would go for months and months without drinking. You couldn't run with the drinking. Then if I ran a marathon then I'd have a drink for one or maybe two days afterwards, and then I'd go straight back into training again.'

'But after I stopped the running, and started full-time work, it was the culture of working away from home to go to the pub and have a drink. I've got a very addictive personality, so I became dependent.'

His mid-fifties – from about fifty-three to fifty-seven – were dominated by alcohol, and his life, including what was left of his family life, began to unravel. 'I thought I could control it, but all the time it was controlling me.' His mood swings worsened, and he began to go on huge, extended binges, one of which, in 2017, lasted three months.

His marriage had been over for a while – 'My family has probably suffered more from my drinking than I have' – and although he had a new partner, Ann, living nearby, neither she nor his children nor his siblings nor his brother's wife could get through to him, though all of them tried. 'If it's not in your head, you're not going to do anything about it.'

In those last months, he was drinking a bottle of vodka a night. 'Pubs were too expensive. I'd just sit at home.' As for running: 'Zero. Not a step.'

Eventually, Ann dragged him, almost literally, to a health clinic. He was close to death – and tests revealed that alcohol abuse wasn't his only problem. A rogue thyroid gland had been taking calcium from his bones and pumping dangerous quantities of it into his bloodstream. The resulting condition, hyperparathyroidism, is often associated with mood swings, depression, muscle fatigue and low energy levels – although the long-term effects are worse. But it is easily fixed. Tommy was put on a drip and admitted to hospital, the offending gland was removed, and within days he was starting to feel better. A few weeks later, on 3 September 2018, he stopped drinking for good.

That's how things stood the last time I spoke to him, anyway. You can never be altogether sure with alcohol, and Tommy is wise enough to know this. But he also knows that his post-alcohol years have been the most astonishing of his athletic life.

Within a fortnight of emptying his last bottle, he was running for Ireland again, in a half-marathon in the World Masters Championships in Málaga. 'My time was the worst I've ever done – eighty-six minutes – but we still won a team bronze medal.' It was just the boost he needed. He was ready to start having dreams again.

By 2019, they were starting to come true. That April, he ran 2:30:15 in the Rotterdam Marathon, the fastest ever by a fifty-nine-year-old. Further motivation came from the fact that he had begun to share his running dreams with his thirty-four-year-old son, Eoin, who, despite being a newcomer to the sport, was showing signs of sharing his father's natural talent. The previous September, in Belfast, the two of them had narrowly failed to break the world record for a parent-and-child pairing in a half-marathon. But Eoin was improving all the time, so there was reason to hope that the best was yet to come.

That October, the two of them went to Germany for the Frankfurt Marathon, with the specific goal of a world-record combined time for a parent-and-child pairing. Eoin struggled towards the end, and was disappointed with his personal best time of 2:31:20, but for Tommy the race could hardly have gone better. His time, 2:27:52, was his fastest for twenty-one years, 5 minutes faster than his 1992 Olympic performance in Barcelona, and more than

2 minutes faster than the single-age world record (i.e. for a fifty-nine-year-old) he had set six months earlier. As for their joint target, a combined time of 4:59:22 sent them straight into the *Guinness Book of World Records*, beating the previous record by nearly 3 minutes.

It was, says Tommy, 'the achievement in running that means most to me'. But that didn't stop him from setting his sights on a fresh target. In January 2020, he turned sixty. The stage seemed perfectly set to establish himself emphatically as the best sixty-year-old marathon runner who has ever lived. He also had a more personal target. He had run several sub-2:30 marathons when he was in his twenties, including that 2:14:46 in Marrakech. There had been a couple in his thirties, too, including the 2:13:59 (also in Marrakech) that earned him Olympic qualification in 1992. In his forties he'd run 2:28:38, in Belfast in 2008. And in his fifties he'd broken two-and-a-half hours four more times, including that 2:27:52 in October 2019.

That Frankfurt record was the one that set him thinking. He was two-and-a-half months short of his sixtieth birthday when he ran that race – and he was 2 minutes faster than he had been seven years earlier. Surely he had it in him to break 2:30 in his sixties as well? And if he did that, he would be the only person in history to have run sub-2:30 marathons in five successive decades of his life.

He decided to go for it, and stepped up his training. He also turned down at least one offer of well-paid work abroad. He was self-employed, and earning enough to get by. Why jeopardise his chances of making another strange running dream come true, just for the sake of some extra money for his retirement? That's part of Tommy's secret: he has the ability, when a target race is imminent, to focus on it to the exclusion of all else. So he trained as if he had been preparing for another Olympics, and when his sixtieth birthday came he felt confident that his goal was within his grasp. But there was one thing he hadn't bargained for: a global pandemic that would see most major marathons cancelled for most of his time as a sixty-year-old.

One by one, his target races succumbed: the London Marathon in April 2020; the World Masters Championships in Toronto in July; the Wrexham Elite Marathon – a specially devised event for a small, select field – in October. Somehow he stuck to his months-long programmes of intense preparation, training twice a day and sometimes clocking up more than 140 miles a week, only to find he had peaked in vain. He spent most of that year in superb shape, and did manage to set M60 world records (for 15km, 10 miles and half-marathon) in gaps between lockdowns. But the marathons wouldn't happen for him. One scheduled event, at the Lisburn Festival of Running in late October, was called off with four days to go. 'I'd done so much training for it,' says Tommy cheerfully. 'I was gutted.'

He wasn't the only runner to experience such frustrations during the pandemic, but for competitive Masters athletes there was a particular cruelty to it all, because the clock keeps ticking whether you're racing or not. Eventually, the passage of time wipes out any gains you can achieve through training.

But Tommy, with two-and-a-half months as a sixty-year-old remaining to him, wasn't ready to give up, and neither were his admirers in the local running community. So a new plan emerged. The organisers of the cancelled Lisburn event would use an already certified marathon route at Down Royal Racecourse (where Tommy had set his 10-mile record the previous month) and stage a marathon small enough to qualify as an 'allowed sporting event' under the rules of Northern Ireland's new 'circuit-breaker' lockdown. This meant a maximum of fifteen people, of whom four would be officials and the rest runners. They initially chose the same day as the postponed Maze event, Saturday, 24 October, but then they looked at the weather forecast and decided to go for Sunday instead.

This turned out to be a mistake: 'The weather on Sunday was even worse than Saturday.' On the bright side, it wasn't raining, but there was a gusting south wind, strong and cold, that would chill the spirits of any distance runner. Tommy was initially too focused to notice. All he cared about was that, after ten months' waiting, he was finally starting a marathon, and he locked into record-breaking rhythm from the very first moments. Soon the local runners racing with him were struggling to keep up. But it was tough for Tommy too.

On a normal day, this would have been a pleasant place to run: mostly flat, traffic free, slightly sheltered on a couple of sides, with the lush turf of the racecourse to distract you on your right (outside the circuit) and the ins and outs of the golf course on your left (inside). But each time the runners headed down what for them would be the home straight, the wind hit them head-on, and with each lap (there were fourteen-and-a-half in all) the cumulative cost grew. 'It grinds you down,' says Tommy.

Lap after lap, he picked himself up, forcing himself

through the wind and refusing to allow even a chink of doubt into his thoughts. He knew that he had to sustain his rhythm and morale to the end.

At first, it worked. After 10 miles, he and forty-year-old Colin Heron were two minutes ahead. But Eoin, on whom Tommy likes to rely for his perfect judgement of pace, had already dropped out, suffering from blisters and feeling unwell. Tommy and Colin surged on regardless, but Tommy was disconcerted. He was feeling the cold, too, and could have been forgiven for losing heart. Instead, he screwed up his courage.

At halfway, Tommy was on schedule for a 2:29:04 finish. After 20 miles, he was looking at 2:29:49. He wasn't struggling, exactly – which was remarkable, given that the then world record holder had been more than 5 minutes slower at this stage. But his margin of error was pretty much down to zero, and he wasn't getting faster. Colin Heron was much too far outside his comfort zone to be pushing the pace: he was already heading for a time 25 minutes inside his previous best. The others were half a lap behind.

With about two miles to go Tommy asked Eoin – who was by then riding nearby on a bicycle – 'Are we still OK for 2:30?'

'No,' said Eoin: 'you've just slipped outside the pace. But if you go now you might still be able to get it . . .' This came as a shock to Tommy, but there was no time to worry about that.

'I was practically sprinting to get on to it,' he told me afterwards. 'I figured, I can't blow up completely in two miles, so I'm just going to have to hammer it and see.' He ran a 5:41 mile, then a 5:35 mile, and for the final 0.2 of a mile he was going at 5:22 pace, which is harder and faster than it sounds – even without the preceding 26 miles. 'For the home straight I was running straight into the teeth of the wind, and it was a long, long straight, and Eoin was counting it down, saying "Sixteen seconds . . . Fifteen seconds . . .", and I was looking at the finish line and it wasn't coming quick enough . . .'

He crossed the line in 2:30:02, winning the race by nearly a minute, breaking the M60 world record by six-and-a-half minutes – but missing out by two crushing seconds on the goal he cared about most.

'I knew I hadn't got it,' he says ruefully. 'I was disappointed. I was so close. Yet at the same time I broke the world record by six and a half minutes.' He laughs. 'Who breaks a world record by six and a half minutes and is still disappointed?'

He picked himself up, determined to try again. But when? His sixty-first birthday came and went, with two more scheduled marathons vanishing from the calendar in his final weeks as a sixty-year-old. Then came the Cheshire Elite Marathon, in April 2021, which caught him just a few weeks after his first Covid-19 vaccination. He had a bad reaction to the jab and lost a vital ten-day chunk of training. His time of 2:31:18 was pretty astonishing in the circumstances, but it was no good for Tommy's five-decade dream.

The rescheduled London Marathon, in October 2021, offered more promise. But Tommy hadn't bargained for the dense crowds at the start, which prevented him from making a final pre-race visit to the toilet. The result was a mid-race stop behind a clump of trees which added more than a minute to his time – and he finished in 2:30:46. 'I'm disappointed,' he said, with admirable understatement, 'but I will go on.'

For the Valencia Marathon, two months later, he resolved to leave nothing to chance. He booked a hotel just 300 metres from the start, to ensure unlimited toilet access, and once again trained like an Olympian. Then came the Omicron variant of Covid, and with a week to go, Spain closed its borders to visitors from overseas who hadn't been double-vaccinated. Tommy, as we know, had had his first jab back in April. But because his reaction to it had been so bad, he never got a second one; and now there was no time to do so. 'It has come back to bite me,' he told me sadly.

His sixty-second birthday came and went, but still he found the inner strength to keep chasing his dream. The next opportunity was the Manchester Marathon in April 2022. 'I will try my best to achieve my goal,' he said, shortly before the race. Yet again, however, it wasn't quite enough: 2:30:07.

To describe that as a disappointment would be inadequate. On the one hand, it was faster than any sixty-two-year-old had ever run before – and within 5 seconds of the sensational world record he had set as a mere sixty-year-old. (In age-adjusted terms, it was better.) What was there to be disappointed by? On the other hand, 'disappointment' is too weak a word to describe the deflation that comes from getting that close, after working so unimaginably hard to do so, for such a long time, and yet still not breaking the magic barrier.

Undaunted, Tommy set his sights on the Belfast City Marathon a month later, but a groin strain forced him to pull out a few days beforehand. All things considered, it was remarkable that his body hadn't broken down in protest some time earlier, but now, in addition to facing the same thankless dilemma as the rest of us (maximise healing time or minimise fitness loss?), he could hear the ticking of the clock growing louder.

Perhaps by the time you read this his luck will have turned. The last time we spoke, he wasn't planning to give up. But time is against him. He is already more than halfway through his age category, and the experience of earlier world record-holders suggests that, in your early sixties, each year adds about a minute to your marathon time. So each time he tries, he has more improvement to find. I wouldn't put anything past him. One day, however, even Tommy Hughes will be too old for such a pie-in-the-sky target.

But he has, I think, come close enough, often enough, to suggest two things. One is that, one day, somewhere, a sixty-year-old man will probably break that two-and-a-half-hour barrier. (Imagine what Tommy could have achieved had Covid not prevented him from having a crack two years before his Manchester attempt.) And the other is that, for the foreseeable future, 2:30 or thereabouts represents pretty much the absolute limit of what a sixty-year-old male marathon runner could possibly hope to achieve.

Meanwhile, a bigger question remains: what is Tommy's secret? It obviously helps that, when he trains for a target, he does so with monastic single-mindedness and intensity. That might mean a run of around 10 miles in the morning, typically at 75 per cent of racing pace, and then the same again in the afternoon, along with as much extra exercise for strength, balance and stability as he can find time and energy for, to compensate for ageing. 'I do a lot of sit-ups, press-ups, and I've got a wee multi-gym in the garage, and I use it. I do a bit of skipping, I've got a punch bag and I do a bit of that, and I'm doing a lot of cycling and swims, cardio training, things like that.' He also uses a foam roller to reduce muscle stiffness and thinks carefully about nutrition, from his daily glass of beetroot juice to his hard-core programme of carbohydrate bleeding and loading in the days leading up to a major race.

The sheer quantity of work may help explain why, in the twenty-seven-year gap between his first 'retirement' (at thirty-two) and his Rotterdam record (at fifty-nine), Tommy's athletic performance declined by only 11 per cent, or about 5 per cent per decade. (Usually, after the age of thirty-five, a decline of 7 to 10 per cent per decade is expected.) The previous marathon world record-holder in Tommy's age group, Yoshihisa Hosaka, experienced a similarly reduced rate of decline, but kept up an equally relentless training regime without a break for decades, while racing four or five marathons a year. In his sixties, however, Hosaka began to slow down more noticeably; and, when the coronavirus pandemic began, around the time of his seventieth birthday, he stopped running altogether. Tommy, by contrast, has repeatedly enjoyed extended breaks from serious training, notably between the ages of thirty-two and forty-eight. Has he achieved what he has done in spite of these rests, or because of them?

The question is currently unanswerable. There simply aren't enough athletes of Tommy's age and calibre for meaningful comparisons to be possible. But that doesn't make him any less fascinating to sports scientists. A team led by Dr Romuald Lepers of the French National Institute of Health and Medical Research (INSERM) first invited Tommy in for tests at Liverpool John Moores University after his headline-making performance in Rotterdam in April 2019. Their interest redoubled when they heard about his father-and-son marathon ambitions, and Tommy was invited back with Eoin for further studies. The pair's training was then monitored for the final two months before the Frankfurt marathon, and the team also analysed the two runners' pacing and nutritional strategies in the race itself.

The really remarkable finding was Tommy's ability to sustain something close to maximum effort for a long time. Measurements in the laboratory, and in the race itself, suggested that Eoin could sustain a VO_2 max of 84.5 per cent, which is pretty much what you'd expect from a very good marathon runner trying his hardest. But Tommy, extraordinarily, could sustain 90.9 per cent. This was right at the outer limits of what is considered scientifically possible, but it tallied with what had been observed in Gene Dykes. As for what it meant: one theory is that the best older athletes may struggle to reach their absolute limits in laboratory conditions – and thus generate VO_2 max figures that are lower than their real maximum. (This is supported by Tommy's surprisingly low lactate reading – 5.7 mmol/L – when he finished his run-to-exhaustion test on the treadmill.) There is, however, another possibility: that the very best older runners have some little-understood ability to run closer to their limits than younger runners.

How they do so remains a mystery. Maybe it's the sheer

volume of their training. Maybe it's a physical resilience, inherited or acquired, that allows them to train or race at a level that would cause others to break down. Maybe it's just age. Or maybe it's a less tangible quality, which in Tommy's case I can only define as 'heart'.

Many of us drift through our sixties sadly, pining for our lost youths, but Tommy is delighted to be where he now finds himself. He is driven: otherwise he could not train as he does. And he has an intelligent, well-informed sense of how his training achieves its effects. But beyond that he isn't too bothered by the science of his physiological limits. He checks his resting heartbeat every morning (forty-four beats per minute, usually), to make sure he isn't sickening. If he isn't, he 'goes for it', in the simple faith that, when he does, anything is possible. As for discouragements, he keeps them in perspective. He knows that his running achievements are just one manifestation of the much bigger achievement of being sober; and his gratitude for this fills his days with energy. He can't remember when he last felt so human and alive.

This is a quality that cannot be measured in a laboratory: a mixture of courage and optimism that succeeds by daring to risk failure, that bounces back from each disappointment with renewed hope, and that always believes that a little bit more is possible. In Tommy's case, it probably is. It just hasn't happened yet.

'The way I think,' he concludes cheerfully, 'I still haven't finished my career yet. It's actually only started.'

11

Strong and balanced

For most of us, the precise percentage points of Tommy Hughes's physiology have limited relevance. We're never going to run the way he does, because we lack his talent. Yet the invisible enemy he's fighting – the force which, other things being equal, adds a minute a year to his marathon time – is the same for everyone. Age diminishes us as runners. It is worth understanding how.

Here are just a few of the more obvious things we're up against.

(1) From middle age onwards, your muscles start wasting away. It's like being a snowman in a thaw. If you carry on training with exactly the same intensity and variety from the age of fifty to the age of eighty, you can still expect to suffer from steady loss of muscle mass – at a rate of between 1 and 2 per cent per year – and muscle strength – typically from 1.5 per cent to 5 per cent. By the time you're seventy, your peak power output (PPO) is likely to be 25 per cent less than it was when you were forty, while by eighty your muscle mass could have shrunk by 40 per cent. And that's assuming that you haven't reacted to the shrinkage by easing off on your training.

(2) Simultaneously, but additionally, you will be experiencing a significant loss of lung function. There's some disagreement about the precise degree of loss that's inevitable, but the conventional view is that your maximum oxygen uptake (VO_2 max) declines by between 7 per cent and 10 per cent per decade; which, again, suggests that seventy-year-old runners have to make do with lungs that are about 25 per cent less effective than they were when they were forty.

(3) Your maximal heart rate – that is, the maximum rate you can achieve through exertion – also declines. The deterioration isn't quite as steep as for lung function, but you can expect a drop-off of about 21 per cent between forty and seventy, with a corresponding deterioration in your running performance.

(4) Stroke volume – the volume of blood pumped with each heartbeat – decreases.

(5) Overall blood volume is reduced.

(6) Your body becomes less efficient at delivering nutrition to muscles – making it harder to rebuild muscle through exercise. Sedentary sixty-year-olds lose muscle twice as fast as sedentary twenty-year-olds, and have to do twice as much resistance exercise to get it back.

(7) As you approach seventy, fast-twitch muscle begins to stop responding.

(8) Aerobic enzymes in the muscle become less effective and less abundant, reducing your ability to fuel your muscles with oxygen.

(9) Your lactate threshold decreases, reducing the intensity of effort you can sustain aerobically.

(10) Levels of most sex hormones decline (think of this as a kind of natural opposite of doping).

(11) Ligaments and tendons lose elasticity and, as a result, become more fragile.

(12) Joints lose their range of motion.

(13) You lose bone density, increasing your vulnerability to fractures and in some cases leading to osteoporosis.

(14) Your immune system becomes less efficient.

(15) Nerve function deteriorates, as motor neurons die and motor units (groupings of muscle fibres and nerves) become less efficient. This results in progressive loss of balance, reduced muscle mass, reduced ability of the muscles to produce power, and, as a result, greater risk of injuries.

This isn't a comprehensive list, but it's more than enough to make most runners lose heart, because this isn't stuff that happens to you because you've let yourself go. It's stuff that happens simply by virtue of the passage of time. It's a fundamental constraint on life, like gravity, and with each new day that dawns it's a little bit worse. Actually, it's even worse than that, because each of these individual manifestations of the ageing problem exacerbates the others. One part of your physiological system stops doing its job properly, so the other parts, which are already struggling to keep on top of their own workload, work harder still in an effort to compensate, and end up failing to do *their* job properly. Cardiovascular exhaustion results in damage to under-fuelled muscles; poor balance leads to accidents, potentially damaging weakened bones; tight joints result in damage to over-loaded tendons – as do weaker muscles or balance mishaps. The one thing that doesn't decline with age is your risk of getting injured.

This reminds me:

(16) the older you get, the longer it takes for injuries to heal.

That's the obvious spirit-breaker. If you can't run at all, overcoming other obstacles doesn't help. And considering that getting on for half the world's runners, in all age groups, suffer from at least one running-related injury in any given year, it is unrealistic for any of us to expect to escape unscathed indefinitely. Instead, the ageing athlete should expect the same irregular lay-offs as everyone else; the only difference being that, as the years go by, the lay-offs grow longer. This means more time for strength and fitness to decline, good habits to weaken and fat ratios to creep up. In effect, you *do* let yourself go. And that means more strain for your weakening body when you try to run again. Of course most people sooner or later lose the will to bounce back.

For the brave minority who persist, there is one crucial item of even worse news. Some time between your seventieth and your eightieth birthday, the real deterioration starts. The causes aren't fully understood, but the mid-seventies slump is one of sport physiology's most immutable facts. You can see it in every one of Steve Harridge's curves, for men, women, runners, cyclists, sprints, long-distance: a dramatic steepening of the gradient somewhere in the eighth decade. You can see it in the 'good for age' times quoted by the big city marathons: in your forties and fifties, the times get slower by about 5 minutes for each successive five-year age category, or 10 minutes per decade; between sixty-five and seventy-five the expected slow-down is an hour-and-a-quarter (an hour and 20 minutes for women). One way of expressing this is to say that age-related decline before the 'mid-seventies slump' is curvilinear, but afterwards it is exponential. Much of this is down to muscle loss, and to the related loss of motor neurons. Even the great German hurdler Guido Müller – who as world-record holder for 300m hurdles at M60, M65, M70 and M75 offers unusually reliable longitudinal data on the effects of ageing on one supremely high-functioning individual – suffered from it; as did Ed Whitlock. The gradient of their declines was gentle and even until their mid-seventies; then it dropped off a cliff.

With so much stacked against us, it's a wonder that any older runner would keep going at all. Yet thousands do; or at least they give it their best shot. That's largely because, for all the difficulties, keeping going is a lot more rewarding than giving up. Even if we never arrive at our intended destination – which we could loosely define as the octogenarians' medals podium – it is just about plausible enough as a long-term goal to allow us to brighten our lives for a few more active years by travelling hopefully towards it.

But there's also a more encouraging reason for keeping going if we can: some of the physiological obstacles listed above may not be quite as immutable as we imagine.

'Look at this,' says Steve Harridge, showing me a cross-section of an individual thigh muscle fibre. 'A histopathologist would look at that and say that's from a young person.' In fact, it's from his eighty-four-year-old cyclist colleague Norman Lazarus, but it's very hard to distinguish from the sample taken from a thirty-one-year-old. It's solid, smooth, substantial and largely fat-free – in stark contrast to the nearby image of a withered, fragmented, fatty fibre taken from a sedentary eighty-five-year-old.

Another chart in Harridge's collection, looking at the mitochondria that allow muscles to make use of oxygen, shows the relative effects of age and activity on mitochondrial fusion (good) and fission (bad). Again, the really serious older athletes measure up startlingly well: their scores are much closer to those for the young than to those for the 'sedentary seniors'.

A third set of images compares the muscle morphology of subjects of different ages; and, again, the cross-sectional area from a seventy-nine-year-old Masters athlete seems as liberally scattered with type 2 muscle fibres as the sample from a fifty-five-year old. What does this mean? Are the serious Masters athletes actually turning back the physiological clock?

'What it means,' says Harridge, 'is that we're still not sure where the limits of inherent ageing are.' The clock isn't being reversed: it's just being re-set, as athletes like Lazarus subtly shift our notions of what constitutes reasonable use of the human body. Harridge likes to repeat a 2,500-year-old saying of Hippocrates, father of Western medicine: 'That which is used develops, and that which is not used wastes away.'

At one level, this is obvious: the more use you can persuade your body to endure, the more slowly it will waste. What is surprising is the degree to which success leads to more success – or at least to reduced failure. All bodies age, but if you train at the highest possible level, the handicaps of doing so with an older body may be much reduced. As a result, that body can train harder and, if all goes well, will age more slowly still. Even injuries might not require quite so much extra time to heal, in an athlete whose cardiovascular, immune and hormonal systems have barely deteriorated.

It turned out that it wasn't just Steve saying this. For the past decade or so, researchers have been reporting similar findings all over the world. In Canada, Mark Tarnopolsky did a study showing that six months of twice-weekly strength exercise training can turn back the biochemical, physiological and genetic signature of older muscle by between fifteen and twenty years. In the US, Andrew P. Wroblewski, of the Department of Orthopaedic Surgery at the University of Pittsburgh in Pennsylvania, concluded that 'chronic exercise preserves lean muscle mass in Masters athletes.' In Japan, Yuko Oguma, Associate Professor in Health Management Research at the Keio Sports Medicine Research Center at Keio University in Kanagawa, reported evidence that 'muscles can continue to strengthen, even in old age, which is contrary to what we believed in.'

Exercise helps. But in that case, given that I had been exercising daily for decades, why did my fragile body seem beyond help?

Manchester Metropolitan University (MMU)'s Institute of Sport, a shiny new four-storey building looming over the Mancunian Way ring-road, might be seen as embodying a coming-of-age for the study of late-life athletes. MMU has a distinguished history of elite sport science;

and of health-related exercise research; and of the study of age-related health issues such as musculoskeletal decay. But only now can all three strands be followed at the same location – which for those studying the effects of exercise on the health and performance of elite older athletes brings obvious benefits.

The Institute is enviably well-equipped. Professor Jamie McPhee, its energetic forty-something director, is particularly excited about the environmental chamber, which can simulate extreme cold, heat, humidity and altitude; about the '3D performance capture hall', whose treadmill 'allows us to record the movement of all the joints in the body while running'; and about a 3 Tesla MRI scanner ('twice as powerful as what you would typically see in a hospital') that is 'probably unique for sport science'. The lure of such machinery, which allows high-quality imaging of joints, nerve cells, muscle, even brain function, is expected to attract researchers from a wide range of disciplines, and the resulting cross-fertilisation should benefit all concerned.

McPhee himself is the product of overlapping specialisms. He started off in sport science, veered into muscle and bone health, then gradually found that, because many of the processes he was studying related to ageing, he was an expert in that too. It led to his involvement in big research projects for the Medical Research Council and the EU's pan-European MYOAGE study of age-related muscle weakness, and he and his MMU team are now world-leading authorities on muscle-wasting and weakness in old age; this in turn has led him back towards sport science, and specifically the study of those who appear to be least susceptible to such decay.

After getting on for twenty years of such research, MMU has a claim to be considered the world's leading centre for the scientific study of older athletes. McPhee himself has been involved in studies looking at such knotty issues as, for example, the relationship between lifelong exercise and 'more homogeneous motor unit characteristics across deep and superficial areas of vastus lateralis' or the relationship between circulating dehydroepiandrosterone and testosterone and motor unit function in young and Masters athletes. He has also led data-gathering exercises at Masters championships all over Europe.

McPhee is currently interested in the role of the nervous system in physiological decline: something that has barely begun to be explored. 'This is really important,' he says. 'It's the connection between the brain and the rest of the body, with signals going out to co-ordinate movements and signals coming in to tell the brain the position of the body in 3D space and what's going on around the body in terms of pain and damage.' He strongly suspects that, in normal ageing, 'changes to the nervous system precede changes to muscle and function,' and he hopes that MMU's state-of-the-art equipment will allow this to be properly investigated. His eyes light up as he describes some of the experiments he hopes to do, involving brain-scanning, muscle-imaging and athletes of different ages, in motion.

You can see why. Like much cutting-edge sports science, however, it may feel a bit remote from the ordinary runner. But McPhee, rather to my surprise, also has two very simple points of practical advice to offer, distilled from those vast reserves of past and future research. Ageing runners, he says, should prioritise two things: strength and balance. These are not the only respects in which we are deteriorating, but they are two areas of precipitate decline, and the chances are we haven't even noticed. They are also vitally important to late-life well-being.

McPhee considers this message so important that, a few years ago, MMU produced an acclaimed pamphlet, *Strong and Balanced*, to get it across to the general public. For a middle-aged endurance runner like me, it makes sobering reading. On the positive side, because I have been training regularly for many years, I am likely to be in a better-than-average state of cardiovascular and aerobic health, and my muscle metabolism should also be very good. But in terms of balance, muscle mass and bone strength, I may not be much better off than my contemporaries who barely exercise at all. That wouldn't have been the case when we were all a decade or two younger, but ageing has moved the goalposts. If I haven't been specifically using it, I've been losing it.

Already, I may have lost 20 per cent of my muscle mass since I was forty. (I'd be more precise, but I didn't think to take the necessary measurements twenty years ago.) Actually, I may have lost more than that, because as a forty-year-old I would have been doing any weight training with heavier weights. As for balance, I'm now no better than an average, non-athletic old person. A fit young person can balance on one leg with their eyes closed for, on average, 27 seconds. The average older Masters athlete – the crème de la crème of the older population in terms of physical function – can do so for just 8 seconds. 'There's something that changes in the nervous system,' says McPhee. 'Even with really athletic older people, they don't read signals coming back from the body until they're big, exaggerated signals.'

When I first tried it, on my left, dodgier, leg, I could barely manage 5 seconds. Weeks of subsequent practice pushed this up to 7 or 8, which was about what I could manage on my right leg. Neither figure was encouraging, because poor balance greatly increases your risk of injury (particularly undesirable if you're one of the substantial minority of older people – 30 per cent of women and 10 per cent of men – who suffer from some degree of osteoporosis).

Targeted exercises won't solve these problems entirely, but they can help a lot. For balance, options include movement-based disciplines such as t'ai chi or qigong, or specific gymnastic movements such as one-legged squats. Alternatively, just practising the standing-on-one-leg-with-your-eyes-closed exercise every day should gradually improve things, in so far as they can be improved.

For muscle wastage, it's mostly a question of regular weight training or resistance training – using as many different muscle-groups as you have time for – plus making sure you have enough protein in your diet. (Nuts have the added bonus of reducing your risk of dementia.) Two or more serious strength sessions a week can also help delay the loss of fast-twitch fibres, bringing significant improvements in maximal and explosive strength, propulsive ground reaction forces, stride length and (reduced) ground contact time, and, as a result, maximum speed. It is no accident that the late Charles Eugster, the British-Swiss ex-dentist who took up sprinting at ninety-five and became a world champion at ninety-six (in 2015), had spent the previous eight years becoming a champion bodybuilder. Muscles are what we run with.

But, says McPhee, there's also a big role for the kind of intense, violent movements that older runners are conditioned to shy away from. 'Endurance runners run for a long time, doing many repetitions of short contractions, and this promotes muscle metabolism. But that's not a stimulus that promotes growth of muscle. Endurance runners typically miss the signal that tells muscles to grow' – with the result that they, and we, waste away. For sprinters and jumpers, however, it's not nearly so bad. 'Sprinters, they send a big signal to the muscles, to activate the muscles really forcefully, powerfully. And that is a strong stimulus for growth, so the muscles will stay a bit bigger and a bit stronger.'

As a further bonus, the big, powerful impacts of sprinting help limit weakening of bones. 'We spent a lot of time looking at this,' says McPhee. 'Bones do respond to impact stressors, and they respond by increasing bone mineral density, which makes them less likely to fracture on impact or from torsional strains.' This ought to be a benefit to all runners, because 'when the heel strikes, that creates stress to the bone.' Yet only a minority of older runners seem to benefit. 'When you compare non-athletes with athletes, you can see the difference with sprinters, who benefit in terms of muscle mass and power and also bone mineral density. But endurance runners do not have those benefits.' Again, the problem seems to be that sprinters and jumpers send big powerful signals with their violent impacts, whereas the deteriorating nervous system simply fails to notice the measured, repetitive movements endurance runners make.

This is unfortunate, because most middle-aged runners are endurance runners – in so far as we're anything. We may not actually run all that far very often, but it's much, much rarer for us to sprint. But McPhee sees this as a positive opportunity for targeted corrective action. 'The first priority is to be active, of course. But if you're already doing that, then it's really worth looking at the detail of how you're active.' And one of the things you can look at is incorporating a bit of sprinting into your running routine, along with some resistance training and some balance work.

McPhee himself is not as fit as he would like to be – 'Work sometimes becomes so intense that I can't train' – but he's active by most standards and runs regularly. And despite being barely into his forties he is already taking pre-emptive action to defend himself against age-related decay. 'I really try to minimise time in the gym, because it's boring. But I do try to include some strength and balancing exercises in my regular daily routine.' He advises me to do the same.

Each runner's needs are different, so he offers broad suggestions rather than a prescriptive programme. 'It doesn't have to be a lot: just a few simple tweaks to your training programme.' For example: 'Try to include some balance exercises in your warm-up or cool-down. And do some strengthening exercises too, especially if you're an endurance runner.' A few sessions a week in a gym, covering a wide range of muscle groups, might be best. 'Or you could just do three lots of ten repetitions of squats – and depending on your baseline strength you could maybe have a bag on your back or a weight on your shoulders.' As for replicating the impacts of sprinting, running on a track would be ideal, but if that's not practical 'you can always just stand on the spot and jump vertically, or even better do some hops on one leg.'

He also recommends incorporating some of this work into everyday life, especially for balance. For example, when you tie your shoelaces, you could try doing so by standing on one leg and lifting the other foot to within reach of your hands. Or, less ambitiously, you could stand on one leg, ideally with your eyes closed, whenever you clean your teeth, or when standing in a queue. It might seem strange at first, but it won't require any more of your time than the conventional approach.

It won't be enough, because some ageing, as we know, is inevitable, and some of the unstoppable processes of decay have an impact on your strength and balance. 'Everyone loses motor neurons during ageing,' explains McPhee. 'By the time you're seventy-five, you'll already have lost about forty per cent of the motor neurons to your leg muscles.' Such losses are associated with muscle wastage as well as loss of balance. But it's still worth taking corrective action, because Masters athletes, despite losing nerves like everyone else, appear to be able to 'rescue' muscles by establishing new connections with new, healthy nerves.

Intense sustained resistance training can also restore muscle mass, even after years of wastage: 'Older muscle will adapt. It becomes stronger, changes metabolism, becomes more powerful,' says McPhee. But the infiltration of fat into under-used muscle, which interferes with basic functions such as the uptake of glucose (and

perhaps also the repair of exercise-induced muscle damage), may be harder to reverse. 'My feeling is that you
could reverse it, but it would take a *lot* of work.'

I can feel my resolve weakening. I would stand a better chance of becoming a high-functioning Masters
athlete if I'd known all this twenty years ago. Instead, I
spent my forties and fifties casually letting myself go,
telling myself that I was keeping fit and strong while my
muscle mass and my mitochondria went to waste. Now
I face many months of intense work just to get back to
what should have been my early-sixties starting-point.
And at the end of each of those months, I will be a month
older.

But McPhee insists that it's never too late. 'Older muscle will adapt,' he says, 'and you're never too old to begin.'
In fact, he adds, even people who have never done any
sport before can 'gain many of the benefits enjoyed by
those who trained all of their lives'. One MMU study specifically compared a group of life-long exercisers (average
age around seventy) with a similar group who had only
started training in middle age. It found 'very little difference in body fatness, bone density and muscle mass'.

For those of us who have been training for much of
our lives, it's hard not to find that last detail disappointing. Yet it's actually quite a useful point for the lifelong
runner to dwell on. What we did in the past is done.
Thriving in later life depends on the choices we make
now. That probably applies to all areas of life, but it applies
very clearly with running. We cannot live off the training
we did when we were younger; nor can we get back any
years we misspent. But we can, if we choose, make a great
deal of life-enhancing progress, simply by recognising

where we are now, starting from there, and heading determinedly in the right direction.

I scraped the rust off my thirty-year-old dumb-bells and (separately) began to experiment with tying my shoelaces while standing on one leg.

12

Starting blocks

I can feel the world champion getting away from me. He's in the lane outside, moving with menacing ease. Flap, flap, flap: his thick mane of pale hair bounces on the back of his head. I'm bigger than him, with longer, more muscular legs. I ought to be gaining. Yet his tidy, noiseless steps lift him easily ahead.

His small white shoes flicker on the edge of my vision. Are they further away than before? I force myself up a gear. My acceleration, compounded by the advantage of the inside lane, surprises him. By the home straight I sense that he is half-resigned to defeat. None the less, I give it my gut-churning best – you can never be sure, with world champions – and I finish emphatically ahead. It's a shame that the stand at Enfield's Queen Elizabeth II Stadium isn't packed with cheering spectators. But I, at least, am flushed with pride.

That isn't quite the full story, as the world champion laughingly reminds me when we've both got our breath back. 'Usually I go faster,' pants Alan Carter. 'And I go over five hurdles on the way.' He's too polite to add that I'm twenty-three years younger than him and really ought to have been able to beat him more comfortably. On the other hand, he is a world champion.

Afterwards, Nick Lauder, Alan's coach, helps us to identify areas for improvement, for both of us. We've been doing a series of 200m sprints, and Nick has been watching closely. He has made videos of each sprint, and assembled stills showing key points in our stride cycles at maximal velocity. The videos are a horror show. Alan's movements are smooth, accurate and elegantly economical. I lumber alongside like a baby elephant, big limbs flailing clumsily. No wonder he can give me a twenty-three-year advantage.

The stride cycle snapshots are more clinical, helping me – or rather Nick – to identify specific shortcomings in my running form. Early analysis suggests that these include excessively casual arm movement (flopping loose and wide rather than pumping tightly, powerfully and straight with high back-lift and follow-through) and a tendency to collapse under my own weight at the 'full support' point of each stride, leading me to waste much of my energy on bobbing up and down rather than powering forward. Subsequent analysis at home using a checklist supplied by Nick will identify a host of other failings, including insufficient extension of the hip of the stance-leg; swing-leg thigh not rising far enough in the drive phase; failure to dorsiflex the foot during the shin swing-out; and excessive shoulder rotation – to name just the most obvious. But Nick doesn't want to 'crowd the mind'.

Quite right. If I tried to contemplate all my stylistic flaws at once, I'd fall over. Even so, it feels somehow reassuring to know that I have so many. Flaws, unlike ageing, can be fixed.

Whether I'll actually get round to doing so is a different matter. I've never been a sprinter, even when I was young and fit. There's barely a fast-twitch muscle-fibre in my body, especially these days. So there might not be much to gain from maximising what little sprinting potential I have. Yet recently I've been gnawed by a strange suspicion: maybe it *does* matter. Maybe improving my track speed, such as it is, is precisely what I need; and perhaps it is even what I want, too. I have known for years that, when I'm not injured, I can plod on more or less indefinitely, if the pace is slow enough and there aren't any irresistibly easy options for quitting. Many older runners can do the same: just look at the back of most marathon fields. As for even longer, slower events: most ultra-runners are over forty, and one in five is over fifty – including most of my ultra-running friends. That doesn't mean that such events are easy; but it does appear that, in later life, a very long, very slow plod is within many runners' capabilities. But a really fast lap or two of the track – a hard 800m race, say, or even a 400m . . . That really would be tough, and way outside my comfort zone. (Even the thought of it makes me queasy.) And if Jamie McPhee was right about sprinters being more resistant to several kinds of age-related decay, I should probably try to get over my acquired phobia of the track.

That's what I've been telling myself, anyway. In fact, I'm joining in Alan's Sunday morning training session mainly because Nick suggested it. He thought I might find it interesting, and, although I haven't known Nick long, I've learnt to trust his judgement. I'm glad I did today, because I have already learnt two lessons. One is that, if you want to be a world champion at any distance in one of the oldest age groups, it might be a good idea to spend a huge amount of time on your warm-up. Alan's

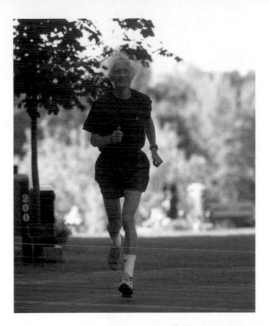

Ed Whitlock, in his mid-seventies, training in the Milton Evergreen Cemetery, Toronto.

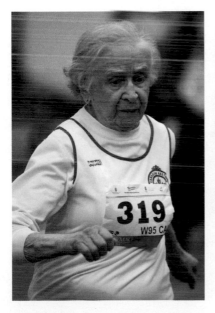

Olga Kotelko competes for the last time, aged ninety-five, in 2014.

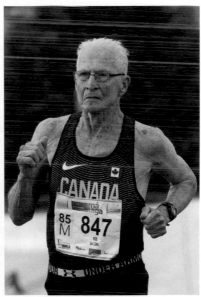

Earl Fee in action as an eighty-nine-year-old at the 2018 world championships.

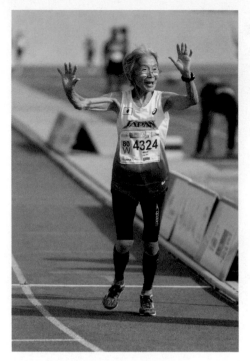

Eighty-two-year-old Yoko Nakano wins one of four golds, and sets an 800m world record, at the 2018 world championships in Málaga.

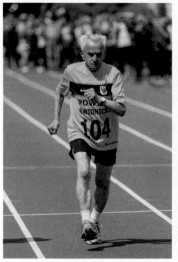

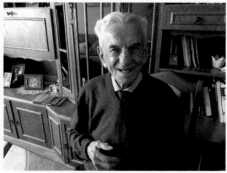

Stanislaw Kowalski sets a European 100m record in Wrocław, four weeks after turning 104; and at home in Świdnica on the eve of his 110th birthday (right).

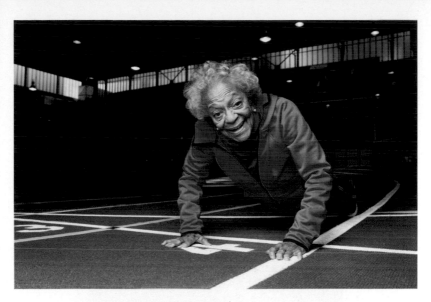

Ida Keeling, 104, shows off her press-ups.

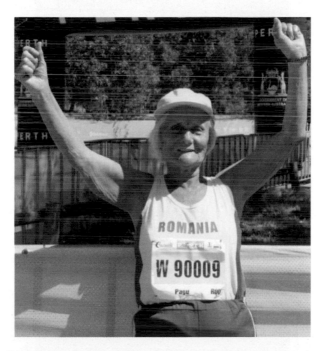

Elena Pagu celebrates one of the two world records she set as a ninety-year-old at the 2016 World Championships in Perth, Australia.

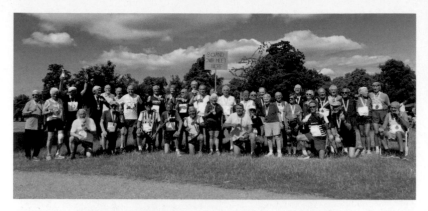

Octogenarian parkrun, Bushy Park, 2021.

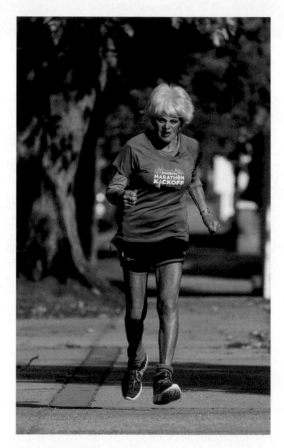

Ginette Bedard, octogenarian marathon runner, in New York.

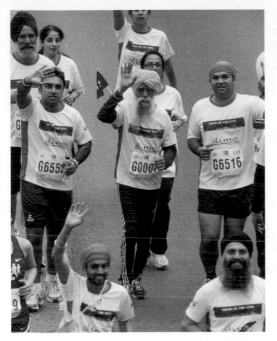

Fauja Singh, centenarian marathon runner, in Hong Kong.

Tommy Hughes, world-record-breaking over-sixty marathon runner, racing in Antrim, Northern Ireland.

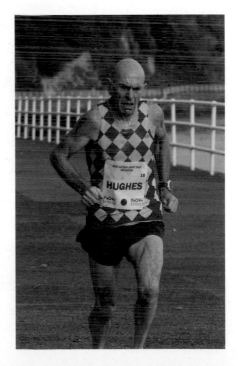

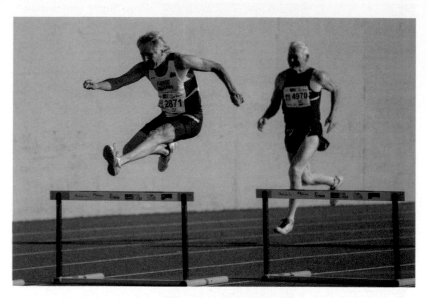

Alan Carter, racing to world championship gold at eighty-one.

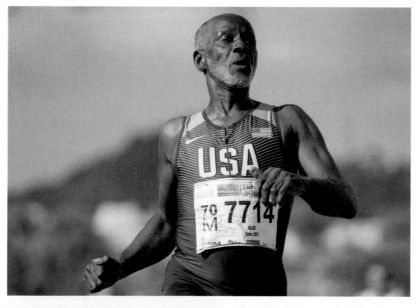

Charles Allie, still capable of running 400m in under a minute on the eve of his seventy-fifth birthday.

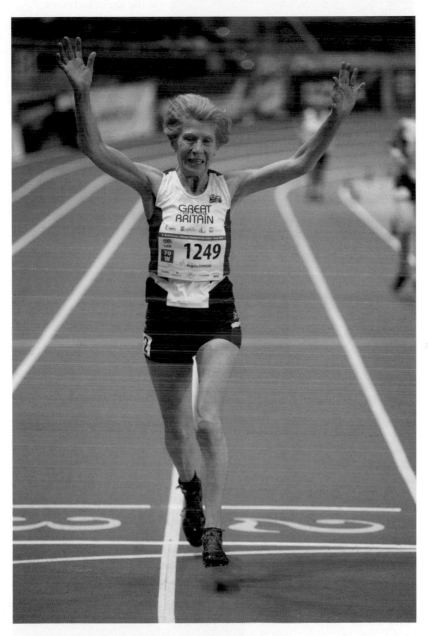

Angela Copson, then seventy-five, wins another gold.

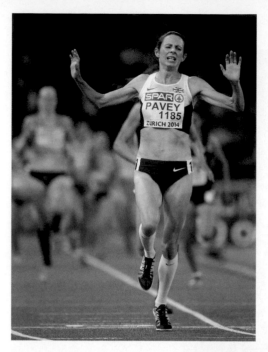

Jo Pavey wins European gold at the age of forty-one.

Virginia Mitchell, fifty-eight, heads for another emphatic 400m victory at the 2021 British championship.

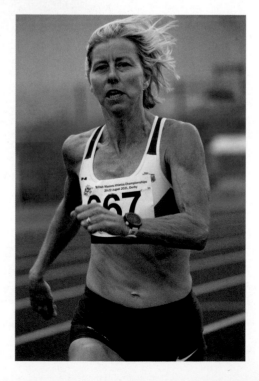

must have lasted an hour, and even now he's still building up to the hurdling stage of his session. Coincidentally – or not – he rarely suffers injuries.

The other lesson is that, on the bare expanses of an empty track, runners' deficiencies – of style, technique or even basic ability – are cruelly exposed. Perhaps I'm being over-sensitive, but there's something about the juxtaposition of Alan's running and mine on video that makes me feel I'm a lost cause.

Nick disagrees. Despite my shortcomings, he points out, in some respects my body positions are closer to the ideal than Alan's. My main good point is an upright torso; Alan tends to lean forward. ('But he's twenty years younger than me!' objects Alan.) Nick has doubts about Alan's back-lift, too: 'I'd instinctively prefer it if he didn't lift his heels so much behind him.' And yet, he concedes, 'It's obviously working for him.' This highlights a harsh truth. Alan is a world champion partly because he is generously endowed with those basic athletic foundations that Nick categorises as physical 'competence' but other coaches sometimes refer to as 'the ABCs' (i.e. agility, balance and co-ordination). He is, in other words, a born athlete. I'm not.

Does it matter? Yes. As Nick points out: 'If you're putting the body in the wrong place, that strains the muscles, which can lead to injury.' But nobody's perfect, and imperfections can, if you choose, be addressed. But the main thing he wants me to take from today is not what I can't do or shouldn't do but, instead, a vivid feeling of what I can do, and what I might do in future. He likes the athletes he trains 'to feel a little bit taller each time'. And the strange thing is, it's working.

Part of this comes from the simple thrill of sharing the

track with a proper, pedigree athlete: a world champion. I suspect this was part of Nick's plan. But I'm also excited by Alan's backstory. He wasn't always a champion. On the contrary, his progress to the summits of Masters sport has been slow, painstaking and, at times, highly instructive.

He joined his first athletics club as a sickly twelve-year-old, in the East End of London in the late 1940s. His mother discouraged him, blaming his recurrent chest problems (later diagnosed as asthma) on his insistence on running everywhere. But Alan couldn't stop. 'It was my first love,' he tells me.

The club welcomed him. 'I was small, but I was fast.' He was best at sprints and hurdles but competed at most distances, and kept it up for around twenty years. Then he watched a clubmate in his late thirties finish last in an open race. 'It was 440 yards, and he looked absolutely stuffed, and everybody was giving him a sympathetic round of applause. I thought, I don't want to do that. So I sort of drifted away.'

It would be another twenty years before he rediscovered his passion. In the interim, he started a family, built up his own business (making plastic injection mouldings), got divorced, and began to feel that he needed a new challenge in life. He had kept reasonably fit, playing regular football and squash, so when a friend of a friend mentioned that her father had 'just come back from the old people's Olympics', he was intrigued.

There was a problem, however. 'I thought I was still pretty fast. I played squash, I could out-sprint everyone else at football.' Yet at his first Masters meet he was comprehensively thrashed, and several of the people who beat him were significantly older than him. 'I thought: there's something wrong here.'

He resolved to fix it, and soon realised what a challenging activity 'old people's athletics' was. Gradually, however, his training gathered momentum, and he was gratified to find that, through sheer hard work, he could still improve his performance. 'My first 200 metre race, when I was fifty-one, I did in 26.9 seconds. But when I was fifty-five I did 25.6.' He was in an older age category by then, so he shot up the national rankings. 'I think I was about third or fourth in Britain. But the guys who were ahead of me were well ahead.'

He stepped up the volume and intensity of his training and set himself progressive targets: first to reach a national final, then to win a medal, then to win a gold medal, then to do all those things at European level and finally at world level. He went to his first world championships, in Buffalo, NY, when he was fifty-eight. He lost both his heats, but it felt like a dream come true. 'It was wonderful: a magical world, running on a proper university track.' His grey eyes shine. 'I was hooked.'

He came home reasoning that, if he kept progressing, he might one day challenge for a medal of his own. It worked well at first, especially when he branched out from short sprints into 400m and his old favourite, hurdling. Then, he says, 'I reached a sticking-point. I sort of held my form until I was sixty, but then in my sixties I started to slow down. I pushed myself harder and harder, but it just didn't happen.'

My ears are pricking up.

Alan looked for the root of the problem. It wasn't an easy journey: it would take him fifteen years to become a world champion. But once he felt confident that he was on the right path – and that improvement, however elusive, was possible – the time and effort seemed justified.

The secret, he says, is to 'train smarter, not harder' – a phrase he credits to the sports psychologist and multiple Masters sprint champion Steve Peters, whom we'll be meeting in due course. Alan met him for the first time in Buffalo, but he didn't discover Peters' training philosophy until many years later – and, in the meantime, continued to train mostly hard, not smart. He accumulated tips from more successful contemporaries, but struggled to let go of his core belief that the key to success is hard slog. When his times were disappointing, he upped the volume of his training. It didn't work. 'I'd be training harder and harder and harder, putting in more reps, over a longer period of time, feeling knackered, and going back the next day, and I'd come away thinking, "Ah, that's done me good!" And then I'd go and race, and I'd got slower . . .'

Gradually and reluctantly, he accepted the idea that less might be more, with much of his conversion taking place in the run-up to the 2007 World Masters Athletics Championships in Riccione, Italy. These took place a couple of months after Alan's seventieth birthday, so theoretically he was in a good position to do well. But only if he trained right. He had worked out that his best chance of running a suitably world-class time in Riccione was in the 400m. But even that was a longer shot than he had hoped. 'Later in life,' he explains, referring to a challenge that we've already encountered in connection with Charles Allie, 'if you can run 400m in the same time as your age, that's regarded as quite acceptable. Well, that seemed like a good thing to aim for. I'd run 67.3 when I was sixty-seven, and so although I hadn't done it since then, I thought I could.' Two months before the championships, he found a suitable practice race: an open race in Bedford for vets of all ages. It didn't go as he'd hoped. 'I was the oldest in the race, and after 300m I nearly walked off the track. I felt so bad. I staggered on, because I had to get a time, but my time was eighty-four seconds.'

For a man hoping to run that same distance in 70 seconds, that left two choices: accept that he wasn't up to it, or find a way of shaving 14 seconds off his 400m time in two months. 'I remembered that my son had given me a book for Christmas, called *The Complete Guide to Running: How to be a Champion from 9 to 90*, by a Canadian athlete called Earl Fee. So I started reading, and it was life-changing.'

Alan deftly boils down Fee's weighty volume to three sentences: 'From about the age of fifty-five, and certainly beyond sixty, your body can't take the volume of training any more. But it can take the intensity. So you stick with the intensity, but you reduce the volume.'

Like most ageing athletes, Alan had been doing the opposite. The worse his times, the longer and more frequent he would make his sessions, which, as a result, became less intense. And that formula had made him a plodder. 'I thought, this guy knows what he's talking about. He's about eight years older than me, and he's won world championships and holds world records.'

The effects were remarkable. Alan applied Fee's core principles to his own training programme, limiting his most important track sessions to once a week – and trimmed his 400m time by more than 13 seconds in a matter of months. At the championships in Riccione, he ran 70.80 in his semi-final, followed by 71.41 in the final. He didn't win anything, but he did make three finals (400m, 200m and 300m hurdles), and he came back with the certainty that, if he kept on training smarter, there was still plenty of scope for improvement.

Subsequently, like Fee, Alan devoted himself increasingly to hurdles, which is arguably the most demanding discipline of all for older runners, especially if, like both men, you specialise in what is known as the 'long hurdles'. For younger athletes, that means the 400m hurdles: ten 84cm obstacles distributed over a full lap of the track. Some call this event 'the man-killer'; others reserve that tag for the plain 400m, before the hurdles have been added. What's beyond dispute is that both events require an agonising combination of anaerobic and aerobic effort; and the older you get, the worse that agony gets. No human being can run anaerobically for more than 35 to 40 seconds, so even without hurdles, the world-record-level Olympic elite have to finish each 400m race with a few seconds of desperate aerobic hanging-on, with excruciatingly high lactate levels in their bloodstream. But the older and slower you get, the longer that late-race purgatory lasts – causing some to argue that the over-sixties should race just 300m in the non-hurdle version of the one-lap event, in case they are tempted to push themselves to the point of dangerous physical breakdown. This remains a minority view, however, and in practice the oldest 400m runners just treat the race as a middle-distance event.

The ordeal is no less agonising with the 400m hurdles, but the hurdles increase both the time and the work required, with the obvious additional danger that extreme physical exhaustion will cause loss of power and co-ordination for an unfeasibly high proportion of the race, exposing old hurdlers to an unacceptably high risk of injury. Age-related stiffness exacerbates the problem, as athletes lose their ability to raise their trail leg to a fully horizontal position. As you move up through the Masters age groups, therefore, the hurdling events are modified. The 400m hurdles becomes the 300m hurdles for the over-sixties, and the 200m hurdles for the over-eighties, and the height and number of the hurdles is progressively reduced. So Alan has progressed from hurdling ten 84cm obstacles over 400m at fifty-nine to seven 78.2cm obstacles over 300m at sixty and then, twenty-years later, five 68.5cm hurdles over 200m from eighty onwards. There are comparable reductions for women, and for what most of us think of as the 110m hurdles (the 'short hurdles'). In each case, the reductions are just enough to make the events viable, but not less brutal.

Most of us are happy to get through life without exposing ourselves at all to such intense, avoidable pain, whatever its precise form. Others cannot resist the challenge, and Alan was quickly hooked. He was good at it, too. He won his first British championship gold at the long hurdles in 2009 (as an M70), and his first European gold in 2012 (as an M75). 'I thought, this feels good. So what can I do if I really train for it?'

By now he had struck up a friendship with Nick, who sometimes trained with him and would eventually become his informal coach. Nick is thirty years younger, with much less experience. A fellow sprinter, he didn't become a runner until he was nearly thirty-five and has done almost all his racing as a Master. He is not yet a world-beater, but he does have one European medal (a relay bronze) and has reasonable hopes of achieving more in future, thanks to a thoughtful, patient approach that he deploys to great effect as a coach. His successes include the late Charles Eugster, whom Nick helped to become a world-record-breaking sprinter in his nineties.

Nick now mentors several successful Masters athletes in the Enfield area, with Alan as his star pupil, and his penchant for cool analysis – 'I enjoy my spreadsheets' – makes him a good complement to the more driven Alan. In 2012 the partnership was still young, but as Alan started doing more hurdle-specific training, Nick's contribution became crucial; as it still is. During our training session, Alan's stride pattern is initially all over the place, and he can barely get his lead leg over the hurdles. A few reassuring words from Nick make all the difference. It is no surprise the partnership has thrived.

In 2013, at Porto Alegre in Brazil, Alan won his first world title. It was his fastest time for 300m hurdles as an M75 (57.28 seconds), and a photograph of his triumph made the front page of the local paper. His son bought every copy at the airport.

Even in his eighties Alan has continued to strive for further improvement while age keeps exerting its downward pressure. Sometimes age seems to be winning: the 2015 world championships were a big disappointment. But between the 2017 European championships in Denmark and the 2018 world championships in Spain, he aged by a year (obviously) but improved his long hurdles time by half a second. 'Often it's a question of what else is happening in his life,' says Nick. 'In 2015 Alan had a few personal things going on.'

These days, however, he is fully focused on being a world-beater. His main worry when we met was that his next big challenge, the 2022 world championships in Tampere, Finland, was due to start the day before his eighty-fifth birthday. This meant that, for the entire tournament, he would count, for medal purposes, as an M80 and not an M85, even though he would be eighty-five for his actual races – unless he could persuade the powers-that-be to make the rules more flexible. Otherwise, he explained, he would just have to forget about medals and focus on setting an M85 world record. (For records, all that matters is your age on the day.) 'I can't expect to beat all the eighty-year-olds,' he said matter-of-factly.

Such goals are rarely far from his mind, even when he's away from the track. He eats and drinks very carefully, for example: 'You have to watch your fat intake, sugar intake, salt intake, drink lots of fluids, and things like that.' And he spends a lot of time weight-training: 'I've got my own set of weights at home – dumb-bells, bar-bells, things like that – and another set at the factory.'

But it's not just about hard work. In fact, one of the things I notice most about Alan's training is how much time he spends *not* working. After each of our sprints, I'm as rested as I'm ever going to be within a minute or two of stopping. Alan allows himself five or six minutes before flinging himself into a fresh sprint with the same intensity as before. This, it seems, is a crucial part of training smart in later life: longer recovery intervals, both within and between training sessions. 'Steve Peters is another one who's famous for his long recovery

intervals,' says Nick. 'Recovery is still the most underesti-
mated part of training.'

Increasingly, and unexpectedly, I feel myself resolving
to use Alan as a role model. It's not that I could ever hope
to do anything like what he does on the track. It's just
that – well, compared with this, the long, slow distance
events I'm used to feel rather tame. Anyone can do an
ultra-marathon, I say to myself glibly, but imagine being
tough enough to run 400m in less than your age . . . That
would be *real* late-life running.

I am of course kidding myself. I'd be pushed to run
400m in less than Alan's age (and ultras are anything but
easy). But the point remains: Alan is a startlingly good
athlete, who has found a way of fighting back against ageing. I am particularly struck by his positive, can-do
attitude. When he encounters problems, he looks for solu-
tions and expects to find them. Sometimes, especially after
an end-of-season break, his hurdling is compromised by
lack of confidence. 'I look at them and think, "They've got
higher. Can I really jump over that?"' So he has made himself some lightweight, adjustable plastic hurdles – which
he assembles, rapidly, as we talk. For the time being, they
are lower than a 'real' hurdle. When he's got his confidence
and rhythm back, he'll raise the bar.

I suppose you might expect such positivity from someone who built up his own plastics business from nothing
and still runs it at the age of eighty-four. But that's what's
so impressive: he defies preconceptions of what old age
should be. There's an energy in the way he holds himself,
and a disconcerting confidence that, if he takes the appropriate action, he can achieve the outcomes he desires.

That's what I'd like to emulate: not the hurdling prowess, but the undimmed inner flame.

Alan attributes his continuing brightness to the fact that he is still working. 'When people retire,' he says, 'they lose their zip. Everything becomes a big thing for them. But I don't feel any different. I'm still looking ahead.'

'Alan can be very hard on himself sometimes,' says Nick. 'But he's still living his passion, and that counts for a lot. Actually,' he adds, 'there are a lot of people in Masters athletics who are like that. But you've probably noticed that already.'

13

The art of smart

I wasn't sure if Steve Peters would have time to talk to me. He is much in demand. Many people seek his advice in connection with his extraordinarily successful work as a sports psychologist for elite British cyclists and, more briefly, for the England and Liverpool football teams and the snooker champion Ronnie O'Sullivan. Others admire the Middlesbrough-born 'mind mechanic' for his best-selling mind-management book, *The Chimp Paradox*, and for the influential consultancy, Chimp Management, that it spawned. He tends to have several other high-powered roles too, at any given time, in academia and sport: for example, as Chair of the WMA Anti-Doping and Medical Committee. But I wanted to talk to him about his life as a world-beating late-life sprinter.

I didn't expect this to take very long, because Peters doesn't like to waste time. He has been spectacularly successful in Masters athletics, yet his running habits are minimal. His achievements – which include gold medal trebles (100m, 200m, 400m) at three different world championships, and British and European records in age groups from M45 to M65 – are based on barely 15 minutes' running a week.

It sounds bonkers, but it's true. In fact, when I

eventually caught up with him, he had been doing even less. The coronavirus pandemic prompted him to give up running altogether for nearly two years, since he hates to train anywhere but on an athletics track and all the tracks were closed. But even as he began to pick up his training again afterwards, he was sticking to the same ultra-low-volume approach.

A typical Peters session – assuming that he is in full championship-focused training – might involve no more than 1,200m of running altogether, including warm-up. The warm-up would include a 400m jog, plus a bit of gentle stretching and some activating leg-lifts. Then might come three 100m sprints, separated by around 15 minutes' rest. The slowest might take around 15 seconds, these days. By the third, he'd be trying to break 12. Then he would take a full half-hour's rest, before doing one flat-out long sprint of either 300m or 400m (usually 300m these days). And that, literally, is it.

Repeated three times a week, when he's fit, this amounts to well under a quarter of an hour of actual running per week, including warm-ups. He was doing slightly less, when we spoke, as he tried to rebuild from that two-year lay-off. But to speed his return he was also doing a weekly multi-gym session. However, he told me apologetically, the whole session – involving quadricep extensions and hamstring curls– 'only takes me three minutes'.

Is this what smart training looks like? 'It works for me,' he said. 'There wasn't any science behind it. I guess I work with the principle that you work with what works for you. So I train hard, quality sessions. I don't like sub-maximal work. I only sprint. I just work with what my body's telling me.'

The way he tells it, most of his success has been achieved by accident. He was a decent athlete in his student days but didn't stick with it. He started his working life as a maths teacher, retrained as a doctor, worked for twenty years as an NHS psychiatrist (including twelve years with very disturbed patients at Rampton Special Hospital), then drifted into advising British Olympians for the first time about twenty years ago. This 'escalated'. Within three years he found himself doing sport psychology more or less full time, and then put some of his thoughts into a book, whose core message (grossly over-simplified) is that part of the human brain is a 'chimp mind' which, if we do not make friends with it and learn to manage it with our rational mind, will hijack our thinking at crucial moments and cause us to react in disastrously over-emotional ways. Many elite sportsmen and women have benefited from these insights.

He stumbled into running, too. He was helping out as a judge at a local athletics meet when a member of a 4x100m relay dropped out at the last minute. Someone persuaded him to borrow a pair of shorts and run a leg himself, so the contest could go ahead. He was so unfit he was sick after finishing, but the watching athletes were impressed by his natural speed and persuaded him to try some training. He did, and enjoyed the improvement; struggled in races against runners much younger than him; and then, at forty, discovered Masters – and his world-beating potential.

Since then, he has hoovered up medals and records, with little visible effort beyond the constant climbs to the top of the podium. You could forgive his rivals for being envious or irritated, but he's modest and approachable, and hard to dislike. In any case, what he does isn't really easy at all. Those short sprints hurt, and leave him drained. 'I've cut back,' he said. 'I can't do what I did.' There was a time, for example, when he would do two long sprints per session. 'I can't do two three hundreds. Not now. I'm nearly seventy.'

Solidly built, with receding lamb-white hair and a jolly face that looks freshly-scrubbed, he speaks quickly and economically, like a man in a hurry. But he chuckles readily, and he is modest about his achievements. 'It's horses for courses,' he said. 'I can't run more than four hundred. I just can't. I can't even jog. If I jogged for a bus, I'd be in trouble. But I do know that if I do three of those sessions a week, I'll slowly build. If I do two, I'll slowly weaken. If I do four, I'm likely to injure.'

You won't find many people who agree with him. Nor will you find many who can beat him. 'I can't tell you how many coaches have said: "If you trained properly, you could do something special." But I think I'm doing all right really.' In any case, he added: 'I couldn't do what they asked me to do. I couldn't do it physically – especially reps at three-quarter pace. I really admire sprinters who can run repeats, but I cannot do that.'

What he can do, and has done as an M65, is break 13 seconds for 100m, and 26 seconds for 200m, and 60 seconds for 400m. I would have struggled to do that in my thirties. So perhaps Peters' approach has little relevance to a plodder like me. Yet there was something about his quiet confidence, and the fact that his training seemed to work so well for him – and that this 'less is more' principle seemed to keep cropping up in conversations with older champions – that made me reluctant to dismiss the possibility of learning from him.

His advice to me – before rushing to his next meeting – was simple: 'Learn your body.' Specifically, he recommends learning to recognise the difference between physical tiredness and psychological tiredness – and to respond to the former by resting. 'I'm a big fan of rest,' he said. 'I like to fully recover. But I also think I've got really wise about recognising when I'm tired and need to stop training.' If he thinks it's just his mind playing tricks on him, he'll drive himself on. But, he advised, 'If you're unsure, rest, because that's better than overtraining.'

Research suggests that the ability to distinguish between physical and psychological tiredness is a powerful predictor of athletic success. I wish I had it. Instead, I realised, I seemed to feel continual confusion as to whether I was tired from over-training or from under-training, or perhaps even both. I was pretty sure I was tired, though. And not getting stronger.

But it wasn't just me. Amby Burfoot had also been feeling the weight of his age. 'I always knew I would get older and slower,' the grand old man of American distance running told me, in the unhurried tones of someone who has given the matter considered thought. 'But I assumed that slow running would be easy. And it turns out slow running isn't easy.'

A former 2:14 marathon runner, who won the 1968 Boston Marathon and still regularly competes in it, the Connecticut-based Burfoot is also a toweringly influential figure in running journalism. He spent over forty years working at *Runner's World* magazine, as editor and writer, and has written half-a-dozen books about running, including *Run Forever*, a wonderfully accessible guide to the practicalities of running in later life. Now seventy-six, he shows no signs of giving up either writing or running. His weekly newsletter for the *Podium Runner* website, 'Run Long, Run Healthy', is a superb source of information from the cutting edge of running and ageing research. And by the time you read this he should have completed his iconic local 4¾-miler, the Manchester Road Race, for the sixtieth year in succession.

'I'd love to be running for another five, ten, fifteen years,' he said, 'but we have to recognise that we might be quite fit but we're also very mortal, and life has a lot of random dice-throwing coming at us all the time.' He still vaguely aspires to be best in his age group when he races, but time seemed to be eroding his excellence. 'I don't have to look very far to find a seventy-five-year-old who's faster than me.' Indeed, one or two of his running friends appear to be slowing down less rapidly than he is. 'It's a little bit of a mystery to me,' he smiled, 'because I actually think I'm training consistently and hard. But we all have very different ageing curves.'

He trains much as he has always done, with large quantities of long, slow distance, often on the very same routes in rural Connecticut that he used half a century ago ('only it takes me fifty per cent longer . . .'). On a typical day he'll do about an hour's slow running – 'an easy six miles at a conversational pace' – and about an hour indoors on his recumbent bike, reading magazines.

Every now and then he'll do some hill sprints, and most weeks he goes to the gym two or three times – although he usually ends up spending most of his time there on a stationary bike. 'I keep telling myself that I ought to do three or four months of a lot more strength training, but I just haven't gotten there, and I'm not sure I will. I've always had this bias that steady aerobic training is more important health-wise than strength training. But it's also because I'm reasonably good at running, but I'm extraordinarily bad at strength training. So I go where I'm comfortable.'

All this felt reassuring. His outlook seemed much like mine, and I couldn't help noticing that he glowed with health. With his bright grey eyes, a neat white beard, and the creased, tanned, thoughtful face of a man who finds happiness outdoors, he looked both wise and wizard-like. Yet his words surprised me, too, because Burfoot is insatiably curious, and intimidatingly well informed, about the general physiology of running and ageing. I had expected his habits to be more cutting-edge.

Instead, like Peters, he happily accepts that what he does is 'just what my body can do now'. After a certain age, he added, 'every single day you're slower than you were before. That doesn't give you a lot of excitement.' He still believes in 'trying to be the best we can be in this crazy world'. But he's less driven by goals than he once was, apart from one thing. 'I would like to keep running as long as I can. And when I can't, I'll walk. The important thing is to move.'

For the moment, he is moving well. He must be getting a few things right. Yet even he suspects that, when it comes to flattening his ageing curve, his approach may be less than optimal. As one of his running heroes, Emil Zátopek, used to put it: 'Why should I practise running slow? I already know how to run slow.' Maybe Burfoot's training (and, by implication, mine) is just reinforcing a natural late-life instinct to run like an old man. Maybe we would both benefit from turning down the volume – and practising running fast.

Burfoot smiled again. 'Sometimes,' he confessed, 'I wonder if I wouldn't get faster by doing sprint training four hours a week instead of doing slow miles. But I haven't found a strong enough impulse to change my system. I'm so habituated to what I do, it's easier to just keep doing it. I do wonder, though . . .'

14

Breaking points

It was Peter Herbert who converted me. He's a seventy-eight-year-old professor of physiology – although that description doesn't really evoke his jolly, muscular, energetic presence – who has spent most of the past decade investigating the relationship between shorter, faster, more intense bursts of training and slower physiological ageing. Based in Carmarthen, in south Wales, he has worked with elite athletes in many sports, including rugby, boxing and cycling. He spent several years as strength and conditioning coach for the Wales rugby team (and many more performing the same role for Llanelli's Scarlets); but, he says, 'Life became so much more interesting after sixty.' His main sporting passions these days are surfing, rowing and cycling, in which he competes with some success. He won M70 bronze in the 500m at the 2018 World Masters Track Cycling Championships in Manchester and, although he prefers to row in the nearby River Towy, he is a former world record holder at indoor rowing. He is also a keen hiker, an enthusiastic sea-swimmer and kayaker and, although he's cut back on it since his knee replacement, a runner.

His academic research – which he started doing at a time of life when most people are thinking about retirement – is equally wide ranging, and still keeps him frenetically busy. Recent projects include a big study on the use of exercise to rehabilitate cancer patients, and a validation study on Wattbikes. But his special subject is the physiology of high-intensity interval training, especially as practised by older men.

He stumbled upon this concept while struggling with his own middle-aged slump. He had always kept fit: in his prime he was a serious rugby player and a PE teacher. But from his late fifties age weighed on him more heavily. He kept putting in the hours and the effort, but 'my body didn't respond.' Nor was it only him. He was a university lecturer by then, and regularly trained with two friends of a similar age. They ran and they cycled, and thanks to Herbert's lab they were able to monitor their progress fairly precisely. It wasn't good. They were still far fitter than the average for their age, but they could see that their training was producing diminishing returns.

Then his two training partners found themselves working abroad for three months, in circumstances that allowed them to train properly only once a week. Herbert continued his three-sessions-a-week regime in Wales. When his friends came home, all three of them tested themselves in the lab. Remarkably, it was the two who had been abroad whose VO_2 max scores had improved, while Herbert's had remained the same.

This set him off on a path of reflection and enquiry that led him to revise almost everything he thought he knew about physical conditioning, especially in later life. Eventually, in 2012 (when he was sixty-seven), he began the seminal study that made his name. Two groups of subjects were recruited, both in the fifty-five to seventy-four age range. One lot were lifelong 'super-exercisers'; the others were sedentary. The sedentary group underwent a very gentle six-week programme of 'pre-conditioning', so they could participate safely. Then both groups did a six-week programme of high-intensity interval training.

The programme was simple. Every five days, they would do a high-intensity workout, lasting 18 minutes. The rest of the time, they would do just 30 minutes a day of very gentle aerobic activity, such as walking or slow jogging. That was all. One of the biggest challenges was persuading the 'super-exercisers' to cut down the volume of their training to that extent. They were used to training hard at least three times a week, often much more, and, admits Herbert, 'Many believed they would see a steep decline in fitness.' But he won them round, and they all conceded that the 18-minute high-intensity session, though minimal, was tough. It involved six 30-second sprints (performed on a bike), separated by 3-minute recovery intervals. Each sprint had to be performed at 90 per cent effort, so the athletes were close to the absolute limits of their physical capacity. By the fifth or sixth sprint most were losing full mastery of their legs.

The previously sedentary group did the same programme. They didn't produce as much power, of course, but they, too, were giving 90 per cent of maximum possible effort for each sprint and had jelly-like legs by the end of it. Many disliked the painful novelty of exploring their physical limits, but they stuck with the programme. And then, at the end, everyone was tested.

The results, says Herbert, were 'overwhelming'. The previously sedentary group had improved beyond recognition, in oxygen capacity, muscle power, muscle mass, fat loss, lowered blood pressure, increased testosterone levels; even reported quality of life. This was gratifying but not wholly surprising, as previous studies had suggested that sedentary people could benefit from high-intensity interval training (and indeed from any exercise at all). But the life-long super-exercisers were surprised to find that they, too, had improved significantly, in most of the same respects. The gains were less spectacular, because they were starting from a much higher base, but they were still impressive. For example, VO_2 max scores improved from an average of 38ml/kg to an average of 44ml/kg, while leg power improved by an average of 15 per cent. Those were big gains, in just six weeks, for hardened athletes (average age sixty-four) for whom big training gains were mostly a distant memory. And they were achieved, as Herbert likes to emphasise, 'by exercising less frequently than before'.

The study formed the basis of Herbert's PhD, which he completed when he was seventy-one. The same year, he became director of the University of Wales Trinity Saint David's newly opened Centre for Health and Ageing. Getting on for fifty peer-reviewed research papers have been spawned by Herbert's 2012 study and its various follow-ups, and his work also forms the basis of the Centre for Health and Ageing's community outreach programme. It is, he believes, the most effective way yet found to improve VO_2 max and leg power (two of the strongest predictors of health span) in previously sedentary old people.

Meanwhile, his research continues to yield dividends, showing, for example, that HIIT can lower inflammatory biomarkers (associated with 'inflammaging') in older men. In addition, a four-year follow-up of the original study found that participants who had continued with the programme had not experienced any of the expected age-related decline in VO_2 max since 2012. Even those who hadn't continued had declined at a slower than expected rate. Results from a ten-year follow-up are imminent.

Strictly speaking, Herbert's core programme is more relevant to sprinters than to distance runners. He insists, however, that the underlying principles hold good for all older athletes. Less is more. More is too much. Short bursts of very high intensity produce greater benefit than longer periods of hard grind. Extended recovery periods are essential. This, he adds, 'is not controversial for older athletes'. Indeed, his one-day-in-five approach has obvious overlaps with the 80:20 training principle advocated by the US exercise physiologist Stephen Seiler (currently a professor at the University of Agder in Kristiansand, Norway). Seiler argues that the way to get the most out of training, even for endurance athletes, is to keep 80 per cent of it in a low-effort 'green' zone, while doing the remaining 20 per cent in a high-intensity 'red' zone; and that the way to get least out of it is to plod tiredly on, as older runners tend to do, in an in-between 'amber' zone.

Herbert concedes that a distance runner adopting his HIIT approach might want to tweak the programme, for example by concocting a package of 'maybe threshold runs of four minutes with four-minute recoveries'. And if I wanted to include extended periods of 'low-intensity, long-duration walking or jogging' on recovery days, to stop me piling on weight, that might not do any harm either. One way or another, however: 'If you want success in stamina-related sports, you have to have a higher level of intensity.' And that needs to be offset by a reduction of volume.

It obviously works for him, and it is hard to believe that he is within sight of his eightieth birthday. He's a lean, well-built 80kg, with 11.5 per cent body fat, and reckons that he is 'fitter than I have ever been'. In 2014, aged seventy-three, he won his first World Masters medal, and he has continued to benefit from his own programme. He doesn't stick to it all the time: it would be hard to maintain the necessary focus. But for up to three months a year, depending on his competitive ambitions, he'll follow a 'very strict' HIIT regime, which 'would involve a lot of HIIT sessions and weight training, all with sufficient recovery time for optimal progress'. The rest of the time, he 'ticks over', often guided by the weather as much as by science. Cycling, swimming, rowing, running – he thinks of it all as play: 'fun and not too painful . . . almost like doing the things I did as a kid'.

There is, Herbert believes, more to come. He speculates, for example, that elite, medal-winning Masters athletes might with suitable preparation be able to manage with only three or four days of recovery from HIIT instead of five, in which case 'over a period of, say, three months that would mean an extra nine sessions – maybe resulting in gold instead of silver?' This, he enthuses, is 'a research project waiting to be done. When I am not so busy maybe I will look at that . . .'

For me, on the other hand, there seemed little point in waiting. So I stopped clinging to my familiar routine of medium-paced plods and spent a few weeks trying to stick as closely as I could to Herbert's guidance. The first week was great. All those easy days made life so much easier, and the HIIT days felt like an exciting, invigorating challenge. By the start of week three, however, I could barely bring myself to begin the HIIT sessions. My body knew what was coming.

I stuck at it, none the less, and, just to be on the safe side, topped up the regime with a few anti-ageing extras: jumps, hops, squats. I felt fitter than I had done for years. Better, I felt motivated: eager to embrace the challenge of ageing. Even on the dreaded HIIT days, I felt that I was rather lucky to be doing this, stretching myself further, pushing harder, aiming higher. And then, mid-way through week four, that stabbing pain in my buttock reappeared, sharper than ever.

The problem was later identified as high (proximal) hamstring tendinopathy – yet another diagnosis delivered with the comment that it was probably just a symptom of my age – and in terms of my training it sent me right back to square one. Oddly, however, this fresh setback didn't plunge me into despair. My appetite had been whetted, and I was starting to believe that, one day, I really could get back to proper, goal-focused running.

Only not just yet.

15

Down with gravity

Bergita Ganse had been studying Masters athletes for several years before deciding to have a go herself. The German physiologist had been a decent thrower for most of her life – shot put, discus, javelin – and so, after turning thirty-five, she entered the 2017 European championships in Aarhus, Denmark. She found it 'quite easy', despite having done 'not much training', and came seventh in the throwing pentathlon. If she worked a bit harder at it, she reckoned, she could win a medal. A year later, at the German national championships, 'Somebody else had just thrown a little bit more, and I thought: "If I throw just a little bit further, I'll be the German champion . . ."' Instead, her knee gave way. It has never been fully functional since.

That was the end of Professor Ganse's career as an elite Masters competitor, but she remains a leader in her field when it comes to the academic study of late-life athletics. A physiologist and orthopaedic surgeon, she became interested in ageing early in her career, after dealing with lots of very old patients. Then she got a chance to work in an area that had fascinated her since childhood: space travel. And this, in turn, led logically to Masters athletics.

That sounds absurd, but, explains Ganse, the three

subjects overlap. Ageing, or a process very similar to it, is one of the biggest hazards of space travel. Healthy young astronauts who experience prolonged weightlessness risk symptoms such as atrophying muscles and plummeting bone density – symptoms we associate with sedentary pensioners. If their long space journey involves not just weightlessness but prolonged physical inactivity, their physiological deterioration becomes even more pronounced. 'When you've been in space for two weeks, and you haven't exercised, usually you've lost twenty per cent of your muscle-mass. And the same is true for bone, if you don't exercise or take osteoporotic medications. And the heart shrinks – because the heart is also a muscle – and there are also changes to the blood vessels.' It's like speed-ageing. But Masters athletes appear to offer compelling evidence that even these processes can be reversed, or at least slowed, by intense physical exercise.

Like the sports scientists, the space scientists want to disentangle those aspects of age-related decline that are avoidable (because they're caused by inactivity, poor diet, etc.) from those that are unavoidable (because they're caused by the passage of time or, in the astronauts' case, by microgravity). They want to establish how much of that unavoidable decline is none the less reversible – typically by physical exercise. And they want to establish the optimum exercise programmes for achieving such reversal.

The challenge, of course, is finding the right balance between doing too much corrective work and too little; the problem being that, as Ganse explains: 'It's not just muscle that declines, and the cardiovascular system. There's also cellular ageing, and tissue ageing. Some tissues can't really regenerate any more, so there's more stiff tissue around the joints. Some tendons become brittle, and often rupture in old age. So as well as the decline in muscle function and vascular function, we have these anatomical limitations. People can't move so well any more.' And if I sometimes feel that my moving parts are simply *perishing*, well, that's because they are.

To make matters worse, newcomers to Masters sport are often bad at recognising their limitations. 'People still have their old movement patterns in their head,' says Ganse, 'and they just give it a hundred per cent, straight away, and their body is not able to handle that.'

But athletes who have been doing Masters for a while tend to have a more realistic sense of their limits and, as a result, are less fragile. And Masters champions, in particular, are excellent sources of data on genuinely age-related changes in skeletal muscle, connective tissue, blood vessels, heart function, resting metabolism and bone density; and on the relationship – if there is one – between age-related physiological decline and intense physical exercise. They are also attractive because, in addition to suffering little or no lifestyle-related decline, they are more than willing, in most cases, to push their bodies to the limits of what's physically endurable during testing.

And that's why, for twenty years or more, organisations such as NASA and the European Space Agency (ESA) have been sending researchers to Masters championships. ESA has funded several projects at MMU, and Professor Ganse – who has worked with both ESA and NASA and spent much of her recent career working for Germany's national aeronautics and space research centre, the DLR – has been going to such events for around a decade. This has brought her into contact with people like Jamie McPhee and his MMU colleague, Professor Hans Degens. 'We have an experiment on the International Space Station together,' she said proudly. Ganse is also a visiting professor at MMU, and when I spoke to her she was about to head off to Antarctica to study the effects of exercise deprivation on people 'overwintering' at the Concordia research station.

At the World Championships in Málaga in 2018, a team from the DLR spent a lot of time investigating athletes such as Ian Richards, the seventy-three-year-old British race walker whose exploits at EMAC-Venice helped make him European Masters Athlete of the Year in 2019. 'They did all sorts of tests: jump tests, overnight sleep tests to track your metabolism, everything,' says Richards, who among other things learnt that he has the VO_2 max of a fit forty-year-old. 'They were interested in me because I'd won three gold medals and set a world record.' Richards was so impressed that he later signed up for a distance-learning degree in Sports and Exercise Science at MMU – even though 'I haven't done science since O-level, and my memory isn't what it was . . .'

The DLR have been collecting data from Masters athletes since 2001. The focal points of their Masters Athletics Field Study in 2018 included calf muscle, connective tissue and mobility; arterial characteristics and blood pressure; cardiac structures and function; resting metabolism; vertical jumping ability; and mental state and attitude. But it was all part of a bigger, ongoing research programme, intended to fill out our still incomplete understanding of the physiology of 'pure' ageing. Dr Jörn

Rittweger, the programme's director, had come to Masters by a similar route to his colleague Ganse. Initially a 'humble physiologist' working with the elderly, he had turned his attention to life-long athletes when he was seeking data about the importance of muscular activity for the maintenance of bone – and then to the space agencies when he was seeking funding for further research. But the three specialisms all fed into one another, partly for the simple reason that, as Rittweger said at the time, 'Questions such as how much exercise is needed to compensate for the effects of ageing have not been adequately investigated.'

But there was and is a broad consensus that, in the words of another specialist in the field, Professor Scott Trappe, 'intensity wins'. Trappe, Director of the Human Performance Laboratory at Ball State University in Muncie, Indiana, has led many studies on the relationship between ageing and athletic training on behalf of NASA, and his view – expressed after a landmark 2009 study showing that a seventy-five-year-old who had exercised regularly for decades could have cardiovascular health similar to that of someone in their early forties and muscular health comparable to an active twenty-five-year-old – is that: 'Part of the challenge is the mindset that we need to slow down as we get older.'

Rittweger agrees. 'Whatever you do, you need to increase the component of strength training. But the next frontier,' he adds, is 'plyometric exercises' – that is, exercises in which rapid eccentric muscle action is followed by rapid concentric muscle action, as when you land and take off in more or less the same movement when hopping. 'I think they are better than strength training,' says Rittweger. 'You stretch tendons and muscles, you activate the neural circuits.' Whether you hop, skip, jump or just run downhill, 'you can achieve larger forces inside the muscles and tendons and bones than with strength training'. This has the further advantage of increasing maximal 'stiffness' – that bounce in the joints and tendons that allows you to convert muscular effort into forward motion. Also, says Rittweger, 'plyometric training contains a lot of high intensity interval training, which is really good for your metabolic system. But you don't do it at the expense of endless knee shocks' – as you would from long, slow endurance training.

But public opinion is comfortable with older runners jogging long and slow. The high-intensity stuff still attracts funny looks. Indeed, armchair medical advisers are constantly urging older athletes to ease off. 'You shouldn't do all that running,' we're told, 'or you'll wreck your knees.' (Not true. Non-runners are seven times more likely than runners to need a knee replacement.) 'Take it easy,' we're told, 'or you'll wear yourself out.' (Again, not true. It's taking it easy that wears you out. A classic study of middle-aged athletes by Michael Pollock of the Institute for Aerobics Research in Dallas, Texas, published in 1987, found that, over a ten-year period, those who kept up their mileage but limited their running to comfortable long slow distance running experienced VO_2 max decline at more than seven times the rate of those who ran the same mileage but continued to race.)

There is a little bit of truth in another old chestnut: 'Don't overdo it or you'll give yourself a heart attack.' But only a little. Those who subject themselves to many unbroken years of extremely high-intensity and/or extremely long-duration exercise may, over time, increase the risk of heart arrhythmias. But you do need to tick all those boxes, and the extremes involved really are extreme. 'I did super-insane training for probably twenty-five years,' says Mark Tarnopolsky, who was treated three times for atrial fibrillation between the ages of forty-two and forty-seven. 'I used to run races where it's twelve hours a day, back-to-back for four days. I'd be crapping blood, and riding a line between going blind and just seeing through a little tunnel to the finish line.' After his third ablation, however, he scaled back his activities, and today, aged sixty, he gets by on around 45 miles of running per week, plus 30 miles each of cycling and cross-country skiing and, every day without fail, 240 sit-ups and 240 press-ups. (When I first spoke to him, he had just been doing the latter in the middle of a crowded airport.) 'And,' he says, 'I haven't had a blip since.'

A more relevant point for most of us is that, overall, regular running is overwhelmingly good for cardiovascular health. The tiny increase in risk while doing it is offset by a huge reduction the rest of the time. Runners are between 45 and 70 per cent less likely than non runners to die from cardiovascular disease. It's also worth noting that most victims of mid-race heart attacks are in their forties. (Typically, they are fit men who have reached a stage in life when genetic weaknesses begin to reveal themselves.) If you're still running when you're close to or beyond retirement age, your heart can probably take it.

As for that other favourite of the caution-urgers – 'Do be careful, or you'll do yourself an injury' – yes, there's a bit of truth in that too. You won't trip over a hurdle if you never attempt hurdling. But the risks are lower than you might think. The biggest study I am aware of suggests that healthy Masters athletes have a lower risk of in-competition injury than younger, pre-Masters athletes – the crucial proviso being that you have to work your way up slowly to competition level. That's the bit that's hard to judge – and if Ganse (who led that study) couldn't get that right, it's hardly surprising that I've been struggling.

It seems perfectly possible, however, that the best way for late-life runners to protect themselves from injury – or, failing that, to maximise their chances of a swift recovery – is to train with more intensity, not less. We already know that the best way for older runners to keep up their VO$_2$ max levels is to push themselves. (Another classic study, published in 1984 by Professor Douglas Seals at the University of Colorado, showed athletes in their sixties who did high-intensity training getting half as much VO$_2$ max benefit again as those who stuck to low intensity.) But the picture emerging from today's sport and space-travel research shows how the benefits of intense training have spread through the whole system, improving not just the muscle mass of older athletes but also muscle composition and mitochondrial function. And that's just the beginning of intensity's virtuous spiral. Better muscle composition (i.e. less fat infiltration) makes the muscles more effective at repairing themselves after exercise – allowing a bigger training load. Larger, less fatty muscles improve metabolic function, allowing you more energy with which to train. All this makes your heart and lungs more effective too, obviously, and thus increases your capacity for intense training.

Even bone strengthens and regrows with intense use. 'People used to think bone couldn't regrow,' says Bertina

Ganse. 'But we showed that you can still gain bone mass, even at a high age, and decrease fracture risk.' Even cartilage re-growth can, it seems, be encouraged by regular weight-bearing exercise, such as running, which compresses the existing cartilage with each step, squeezing out waste and drawing in fluids rich in nutrients and oxygen. In each case, however, you need to do the work. It's the high-achievers in Masters athletics who fend off ageing best; and within that group (according to recent research by Samuel da Silva Aguiar and Caio V. Sousa at the Universidade Católica de Brasília), it's sprinters who are slowest to succumb to the late-life acceleration in decline.

None of this is easy, even for the dedicated. Reduced levels of growth hormone and testosterone limit our ability to build muscle. We make less creatine phosphate and, as a result, have less short-term energy for repetitive sprints or plyometrics. And even the most rigorous regime of balance and co-ordination exercises will do no more than slow the deterioration of our nervous systems.

But it's worth the effort, because the late-life runner really has only two available options. You can force yourself up the virtuous spiral; or, by default, you will find yourself going down an equally steep downward spiral. Wasting muscles become less effective muscles, with high levels of fat infiltration and mitochondrial breakdown. Metabolism malfunctions – among other things affecting our insulin sensitivity. Exercise efficiency – the output you get from a given energy input – declines. Bone weakens. We become less and less able to support a heavy training load; and, as a result, we train less, causing our cardiovascular capacity to shrink.

It's the familiar pattern of earthly unfairness: to those that have, it shall be given, while from those that have not, it shall be taken away. But simply deciding that you would prefer to be in the first group doesn't mean that you will succeed. There is much to go wrong – and ultimately there is no correct answer to the dilemma expressed by Olga Kotelko: 'If you undertrain, you might not finish. If you overtrain, you might not start.' It appears, however, that undertraining is a bigger danger. You just need to over-train sensibly; or, failing that, luckily.

And if that seems confusing, it's worth remembering that there is really only one thing that we know for certain about physical exercise in old age: if you don't do it, you'll decline. Everything else is research in progress.

If in doubt, train. When you can, train hard. Give yourself plenty of recovery time too, but when you go for it, go for it. It may go wrong, people may disapprove, and sometimes it may feel futile, especially if you have no aspirations to competitive glory. But there are still two good reasons to resist the temptation to behave more sedately. One is that a more intense struggle produces a range of side effects – extended health span, greater physical resilience, more mobility, less dependence, more self-esteem – that can hugely enhance our ability to enjoy our remaining years. And the other is that, for many, the burning effort is its own reward.

Sometimes, in sport, we talk about having 'a mountain to climb': in other words, a tough and daunting battle. But struggling against a mountain to the limits of your courage and endurance can often be a profoundly life-enhancing ordeal. Our efforts cannot make the mountain tamer or smaller; yet sometimes we find that, in the despair and defiance of the struggle, we ourselves are changed, and become somehow bigger.

This might be the single most important thing you need to know about trying to be a runner in old age. It's a battle you can't win, but you can choose to go down fighting. It's a bit like running up a down escalator, or – the image that keeps coming back to me – being on one of those crumbling slopes that troubled me in the Lake District. I imagine us standing on a particularly precipitous scree slope, a little way below the summit of a big, steep mountain, and feeling the stones slipping down alarmingly beneath our feet. Gravity dictates that, if we do nothing, we will slide down inexorably towards a ghastly abyss. If we choose, however, we can strike out with all our strength towards the summit. We will never reach the top: the scree will merely slip down faster. And ultimately we too will plunge into the abyss. Yet if we keep giving it everything our net loss of height will be much more gradual. And in those brief, lung-bursting moments of reclaimed time, we can marvel at the power of our wills and the fierce beauty of the summits above us. And occasionally, too, for a miraculous moment or two, we may even shake off the bonds of gravity and age and, very briefly, feel ourselves ascending.

16

Lost time

On a damp, grey, August Saturday, I sat for several hours in a half-empty athletics stadium in Derby, just off the A5111 ring-road. A few weeks earlier, such a gathering would have been illegal, but England was enjoying a brief interlude of light-touch Covid regulation, and those involved were keen to make the most of it.

You could feel the buzz, and not just because of a loud power tool on the adjoining building site. The place was swarming with animated old people: several hundred of them, scattered across the track and the partially covered stand. Some pottered purposefully; others were busily checking kit or equipment. But most just mingled, heedless of the moist breeze, chatting in small clusters with the casual, half-preoccupied familiarity of colleagues catching up after their summer holidays.

There was apprehension in the air as well as cheerful excitement. Something big was obviously about to happen. In fact, you could almost have imagined the scene as a school playground on the first day of term, if it hadn't been for all the grey hair and lined foreheads.

This was the opening day of the 2021 British Masters Outdoor Track and Field Championships. But it was also more than that. For the first time in eighteen months, the hard core of Britain's oldest track-and-field athletes were getting together for a day's shared sporting endeavour. And they could barely believe it was happening.

Delighted greetings merged into a happy cacophony: 'It's been so long'; 'You're looking fit'; 'We made it!' It was a long time since I had seen so many smiles in one place. (Masks were only for the changing rooms.) 'Look at you all!' mock-squealed a new arrival to a female group warming up near the long-jump pit, prompting coos of welcome and laughter. 'They're athletes but they're also human beings,' explained Alex Rotas, visibly relishing her first opportunity to photograph those athletes since before the pandemic. 'For many of them, this is like a second family. And it's been a long time.'

The last such event, the British Indoor Championships at Lee Valley, Edmonton in March 2020, had been notable for, among other things, its failure to spread coronavirus. Other big sporting gatherings that month, such as the Cheltenham Festival or Liverpool's Champions League match against Atlético Madrid, had notoriously turned out to be 'super-spreader' events. But two days of intense indoor exertion by hundreds of notionally vulnerable old people do not appear to have resulted in a single infection. A testament to the miraculous effects of physical fitness? Or mere luck? Either way, the subsequent months of isolation had been cruel, and for the reunited Masters there was sadness to catch up on as well as news about fitness and training. Old faces were missing; murmured explanations told of unscheduled intrusions from cancer, heart disease, dementia, or joints that had simply given up the ghost. Tony Bowman, the popular octogenarian sprinter, hurdler and decathlete, had not only lost his wife to Covid but also recently suffered a heart attack that (unlike his previous two) had 'really frightened me' – to the extent that he now felt obliged to limit himself to the throwing events. None the less, he pronounced today's occasion 'wonderful'.

The races began almost unnoticed. There were more kitbags than people on the plastic seats, and more people chatting than watching. The unhurried announcements on the PA system reminded me of a village fête. Yet the lack of presentational fanfare, like the intermittent drizzle, emphasised the bright enthusiasm of the old men and women taking part and, if you watched, the passionate intensity of their efforts.

I say 'old'. In fact, some of the athletes were less old than me. But even the youngest were over fifty-five, because the younger age groups were competing separately the following day, to help with Covid compliance. So most of today's athletes were in their sixties, seventies and eighties, and the habits of a lifetime still require me to think of such people as 'old'. Apart from me, obviously.

What really singled me out, however, wasn't my imagined youth but something more uncomfortable. I was a spectator. Everyone else was actively doing something: running, hurdling, jumping, vaulting, throwing – or, at the very least, animatedly officiating, or yelling encouragement to relatives or friends. As at a school sports day, the point wasn't the spectacle but the immediacy of personal involvement.

In fact, the spectacle was pretty good, if you happened to be looking. Derek Jackson slashed two seconds off the British M70 record with a 1500m run of 5:08.27; eighty-two-year-old Kath Stewart set a British record (91.84) in the W80 400m; and Lisa Thomas ran the second fastest W55 time ever (7:52.12) to win the 2,000m steeplechase. Barry Marsden dominated the M55 hurdles, long and short; Sue Frisby did the same double in the W60s; and Virginia Mitchell – who had spent most of 2020 unable to train properly because of her damaged heel – won the W55 400m and 800m so effortlessly that she seemed to be in her own separate races.

But you had to be watching carefully to notice such achievements, and not everyone was. Instead, they were absorbed in their own events, or in the efforts of those they had come to cheer. Yet somehow this jumble of disparate individual experiences added up to a potent cocktail of collective enthusiasm and engagement. The goodwill seemed to warm the half-empty rows of damp seats.

It warmed the track too. No one was holding back, and the level of performance was often insanely high: imagine, a sixty-year-old woman running 80 metres, and jumping eight 68.6cm hurdles, in 12.98 seconds . . . But there were also-rans too, some of them far, far behind. In the sprints, starting blocks were optional, and there were runners in leggings as well as runners in Team GB kit. There were even a couple of M60 events in which, had I been running, I felt that I might have avoided last place (although only because in each case the final straggler was limping).

Often the last finisher in a race would take half as long again as the winner, sometimes longer still. Invariably, however, the fast ones would wait on the finishing line (for more than three minutes, in the M65 1500m) to applaud every last runner home. This mutual respect and encouragement is one of the strongest traditions in Masters, and reflects a general recognition that anyone still competing as an athlete after half a lifetime of physical and emotional wear and tear is, at some level, both a survivor and an achiever. According to Alex Rotas, older athletes look after one another 'because they know the crap we humans have to go through'.

'We have incredible unity,' said Virginia Mitchell, 'because we all share very similar experiences. People have been through a lot in their lives, and sometimes if you're all in the same age group you've been through it at the same times: you know, marriage, career, children, helping children through university. There are people in Masters I've literally grown up with.

'Everyone's got a story. They've had some sort of obstacle or health issue, or they've come back from something, or they've had a family loss. Or you go through these injuries and you think I'm never going to get better. And yet here we all are, and we're still doing it. So we love watching everybody else. I think it's great when we see exciting performances, like my friend Iris Holder, who runs nineteen seconds or so for 100 metres, and she's eighty! Great! Let's see that happen. I think it brings everyone together. You kind of think, well, I'm proud of you, because you've got over this, that or the other, and yet you're still achieving.'

It would have been odd if the long months of pandemic hadn't heightened many athletes' sense of life's frailty. They themselves had generally got off lightly: I have heard of only one case of an active Masters athlete who actually died from Covid-19 (the US W80 javelin thrower Mary Roman). But of course the athletes' fitness could not protect their loved ones; nor could it guard against life's random cruelties. Tony Bowman had shrugged off the virus after a couple of days, only to lose his beloved Betty, and he was not the only Master to endure such loss.

Meanwhile, far beyond Derby, the general shutdown of sport and society had deprived many elderly athletes of much that made their lives feel worth living. 'I used to have a positive attitude,' Richard Pitcairn-Knowles told me not long before these championships, 'but with these blooming lockdowns I've not been running much.' 'Some days I feel great,' said Penny Elliott, a leading M75 10,000m runner from Surrey, 'but next time I'm out I have no energy.' Nor was this just a British phenomenon. 'I feel no motivation, no desire,' confessed Denise LeClerc, eighty-seven-year-old *grande dame* of French late-life distance running, shortly before announcing her retirement. 'It's all wiped out.'

Others had the desire but not the opportunity. Jiří Soukup, the legendarily versatile and durable Czech athlete (runner, jumper, decathlete, jockey, skier, swimmer), was shut up in a care home for his own protection and died there, lonely and confused, a few weeks short of his ninety-fourth birthday. In the US, Donald Pellmann, record-breaking centenarian sprinter, jumper, thrower and winner of more than 900 Masters medals, languished in an 'assisted living' home in Santa Clara, California. He had been based there for years, by choice, to be with his frail wife, Marge – and often surprised passers-by by practising his sprints on the pavement outside. But the combination of widowerhood and enforced inactivity sent him into a decline, and he died, aged 105, in June 2021.

'This is taking away time that we don't have to spare,' the American M75 400m runner Bruce Rubin had said to me earlier in the pandemic. 'Some seniors [i.e. Masters] may find they have participated in their last event, if this doesn't end soon.' Even in the best of times, wise old runners know that they have only a limited number of competitive opportunities remaining. In times of plague and war, that last race may be nearer than you think.

Hence the passion with which the athletes in Derby seized this damp day. It may not have been perfect, in its timing or its scale or its profile. But it was happening, and it wasn't long since that had seemed impossible. For most people, therefore, the day had less to do with long-term plans than with seizing an available moment – because who knew when the next such event might come? There was no point in being half-hearted.

The ferocity of competitive striving was unsettling at times, with several runners limping off in distress after pushing themselves a little too hard. One unfortunate M55, the 400m runner John Tilt, had to be stretchered off, after his knee gave way in the final strides of a desperate neck-and-neck home-straight battle. 'His mind was stronger than his body,' observed his friend Virginia Mitchell, distraught on his behalf. Perhaps he should have been more cautious, like me, but where would that have got him? If you don't seize the moments life offers to you, you risk never having tried at all.

That was what made these contests so inspiring. Athletes were pushing themselves to breaking point because they were living their lives to the full – living the current moment to the full – and to do any less would be to waste the opportunity they had been given. Some seemed to find the striving cathartic, and perhaps also empowering. Tony Bowman, for example, bereaved, plagued by heart trouble and not sure if he would ever run again, didn't waste a moment asking for anyone's pity. He was too busy pouring all his strength and competitive spirit into the throwing events – to such good effect that he came third in the M85 discus, second in the javelin and second in the shot-put. In action, his face was contorted with concentration and effort, but between throws he smiled like a boy. 'The important thing', Bowman told me later, 'is that you need to have a go. You've got to put yourself on the line.'

But I hadn't, and it bothered me. Instead, I was skulking in the front row feeling sorry for myself: a healthy sixty-one-year-old (by then), envying the physiological good fortune of athletes who, in many cases, had infinitely more to complain about than me. There were cancer survivors, heart attack survivors, people who had come through terrible loss or accident, and any number of others who with a little less courage might have succumbed to age-related despair. But they hadn't succumbed, and now they were rejoicing in whatever remained of their physical gifts; celebrating life. Bowman, who struggled for breath walking up to the back row of the stand, said that he considered himself 'the most fortunate man in the world'.

Such spirit struck me as remarkable; heroic, even. But my admiration for the brave Masters around me merely increased my discomfort at my own feebleness. I had, to be fair, several solid reasons for not competing: my hamstring, for a start; but also a reluctance to embarrass myself. I knew how good some of these people were: it would have been insulting to ask them to share their starting line with a mediocre athlete like me. Or that's what I told myself. Yet watching these races reminded me of one of Masters athletics' most distinctive features: everyone is welcome. The official Olympic movement has long forgotten its founding ideal: that 'the important thing is not the winning but the taking part.' The Masters have not.

They know it would all be much more efficient if the competition were streamlined with qualifying standards, just as it would be easier for the winners to head straight for the showers. But, really, is making things easy and efficient the most important thing at this stage of life? We are all engaged in the same terrible, un-winnable battle against decay and death. The more allies we have, the better.

That, at any rate, was roughly what I had been thinking before I started chatting with Mike Duggan, a middle-distance runner who runs for Northbrook AC, near Coventry. We had sought shelter from the increasingly heavy drizzle in the shadow of the same tree, and it turned out we had other things in common. Both based in the Midlands, we were both admirers of Emil Zátopek (with whom Mike once jogged, briefly, in his student days). And we both had a problem with our right buttocks. 'I don't know what caused it,' Mike complained, echoing my own thoughts. 'It just appeared from nowhere a couple of weeks ago. I was fine until then.'

We discussed our symptoms and the treatments we had tried. Between us I think we had tried most. But Mike's interest in the subject was more urgent than mine because, unlike me, he was just about to race, in the 800m. Also, unlike me, he's eighty.

He expressed surprise that I wasn't racing too, then went off to coax his hamstring into cooperation with a couple of hours of gentle, patient warm-up. And then, towards the end of the day, he raced, in the 800m. He came second overall, running against three M75s, but first in his age group, for which he was the only competitor. His time, 3:31.64, was 23 seconds slower than the British M80 record, but it was still enough to make him a British champion.

It would be hard to find a more elegant proof of Woody Allen's theory that 'Showing up is eighty per cent of life.' But what gnawed at me as I watched – and again as I drove home, without having broken sweat – was a related truth: that few failures provoke such bitter shame and regret as not showing up. I have spent much of my life being rash while those around me were being prudent, and then wishing I hadn't. But today had left me with a different kind of remorse.

17

The whole garden

Pete Magill is a middle-aged Californian: a former scriptwriter who spent most of his thirties in a haze of substance abuse. He turned his life around when he was thirty-eight, after waking up in a hospital emergency room and being told that he wouldn't live to see his son graduate from high school. Feeling his life in the balance, he remembered the brief promise he had shown as a young athlete and – as so many of us have done in our different ways – healed himself with the help of a patiently nurtured running habit.

He got his health back. He became 'a viable, decent human being in the lives of the people around me, instead of . . . you know.' He also became an astonishingly successful runner. A six-times national Masters cross-country champion, Pete has a string of spectacular achievements to his name, including the fastest ever 5km and 10km times by an American over fifty (15:01 and 31:11 respectively). But he is mainly revered for his achievements as a coach and best-selling author. Based in south Pasadena, he coaches at everything from high school level to Masters level, and has guided the Cal Coast Track Club to nineteen national Masters championships in cross-country and road racing. His 2014 book, *Build Your*

Running Body, was described by Bob Anderson, founder of *Runner's World*, as 'the best running book ever'. If you're looking for detailed, authoritative, practical guidance on training, it might be the only running book you'll ever need.

He seems like a good person to share my running problems with. I have just been doing so, at some length.

'Of course you got injured,' he tells me. 'You didn't do the training.'

But I've been training daily for decades, I protest. I just told you about it.

Yes, says Pete, but what did you do?

'I ran,' I say, thinking again about all those years of casually knocking out the early-morning miles.

He laughs: he has come across many runners like me. 'Just distance running, running easy, doesn't build up the strength you need to ward off injuries,' he explains. 'It doesn't strengthen all of your muscles.' This is partly a question of muscle fibres. Running at a comfortable pace trains slow-twitch muscle fibres, but for all the benefit the fast-twitch and intermediate fibres get you might as well have stayed in bed. Of course we get slower as the years go by. But that's not all.

'People think that when they go out and do distance runs like that, running easy, they're using their muscles. You use your calves, you use your quads and use your hamstrings, and you use your glutes, but at less intensity. But actually you don't. You're using the very smallest subset of slow-twitch muscle fibres in the calf muscle, you're using a very low amount of your quads, and you're using almost no hamstrings and glutes, and the rest of the muscle isn't training. And you won't strengthen your connective tissue enough, because you aren't putting the tug on it, you aren't doing a full range of motion. And then when you go out and you run a race, and you try to run faster, you're putting more force into the ground, and you're going to get injured.

'I tell people this,' he says, 'and they still don't get it. So I tell them it's like having a garden, and you only water a third of it. And then the next day you only water the same third, and then the next day, and the next. And then you say, "Why is two-thirds of my garden dead, when I water it every day?" *Because you didn't water it all.*'

In our twenties and early thirties, he adds, we can get away with such neglect. 'When you're young, you can get away with anything. But not in Masters. Masters is a no-mistake zone.'

That's a shame. I seem to have mis-spent much of the past decade, athletically speaking. 'If I'd known I'd still be running at this stage of my life,' I tell him, 'I'd have taken better care of myself.'

'None of us knew!' he laughs. 'Who'd have thought it? We're in our sixties! I thought I'd be done at twenty-two.'

It's very hard not to like Pete. He has a ready chortle, a lived-in face and a good listening manner. He also has a deep-rooted sense of what is and isn't important in life. The running-related achievement in which he has taken the greatest pride since becoming a Master was watching his son graduate from high school. 'Running gave me my life back,' he says. 'So I'm happy to offer whatever I can.'

But what he's told me so far hasn't exactly raised my spirits. If two-thirds of my garden is dead from neglect, is there any hope for me?

'There's always hope,' he says, yawning into a huge

mug of coffee. The previous day he took his high-school cross-country team to the final meet of the season, and he's still 'wiped out' from the 400-mile round trip. 'You have to adjust your expectations,' he continues. 'Those fast fibres you've lost aren't coming back. But with the correct training you can retrain your nervous system, and build back intermediate fibres.'

So what is the correct training?

The big thing, he says, is to remember that 'there is no such thing as a good training workout. There are only good training programmes. Change is incremental. A workout that's good at one point in the programme might be harmful at another.' That's why people use coaches, to calculate their precise, specific, progress-related needs.

The other key point is patience. 'There are no giant gains, and there are no shortcuts. Training is always incremental. If you want to know how incremental, think about when you get a cut on your hand. When you were a kid it would be gone in a couple of days. But now in our sixties, sometimes you look at your hand, and you think: "Oh, man, I remember that. I did that a month and a half ago . . ."'

The same basic processes of healing – slowed down in the old – are involved when we train. 'You don't get better during a workout. You get better when you're recovering from a workout. You start a workout *here*' – he holds his hand horizontal in front of his nose. 'And then you beat up the muscle fibres and break them down, and tear muscle fibres – you tear myofilaments – and you deplete your muscle glycogen and your neurotransmitters and everything else. And you beat up your connective tissue, you break down bone and put too much stress on it. And you started the workout here, fitness-wise, and you finished it *here*.' His horizontal hand is now down at chin level.

'OK. That's what the workout did. It made you a worse runner than when you started. So the first phase of recovery is to let your body replace those neurotransmitters and muscle glycogen, repair the muscle, repair the connective tissue. So now' – the hand rises to nose level again – 'we're back to where we were at the beginning of the workout. Only it's two days later.

'But the next big mistake people make is they think, "OK, I'm recovered. Let's do the next hard workout." Bam, bam, bam. Two more days. Recover. Let's do the next hard workout. But here's the problem: where do we end up each time? Right back where we started. So why am I training so hard?

'And this is where the idea of super-compensation comes in. I break myself down, boom, boom, boom. Come back up, two days later. But if I then wait one more day, my body goes: "I'm not going let you break me down that badly next time, so I'm going to be a little stronger." So it makes your muscles a little stronger. It makes your bones a little stronger. It adds a little bit of muscle glycogen. And now you're *here*.' The hand is now at eyebrow level. 'So now you do your next hard workout, and when we recover next time we're here' – back at eyebrow level – 'and when we super-compensate, we're *here*' – by which time his hand is where his fringe might have been were he twenty years younger.

You'll have got the idea. 'If we keep doing this, week after week, month after month, year after year, all of a sudden we're off the charts. But it's an incremental process, and you have to be so patient with it.'

Hard-core runners reading this may feel that Magill is spelling out the obvious. But most of us rarely give such matters analytic thought. In so far as we aspire to improve – and most of us do, up to a point – we instinctively assume that we can do so simply by working harder: by running further, or more frequently, or with a bit more welly. Maybe, if running-specific drills or exercises come to our notice and we like the sound of them, we'll add them to our repertoire and give them a try when we feel like it. But there's no thought-through programme: we just muddle forward as best we can.

When we're young, this seems to work. Many of us become better than we expected, and our improvement or lack of it roughly corresponds to our training. Put more in, get more out: that's the basic equation of running. But in later life the formula goes awry, and for those of us who prefer an instinctive approach to an analytical one that can mean big problems. Our running habits – of mind as well as body – become less appropriate to our needs each year. And even when we notice the unwelcome consequences, we rarely change our mindset.

Instead, we tend to hang on grimly to the past. 'This used to feel easier,' we tell ourselves; or: 'I ought to be able to do this faster, like I used to . . .' Or, on the rare occasions when training is going well: 'Right, now I need to up the workload, until I'm back to the kind of routine I used to have when I was properly fit.' Needless to say, the training soon breaks down again.

This isn't our bodies letting us down. It's our minds. It's like being one of those doomed military planners who prepare for the previous war rather than the next one. Pete – picking up where Steve Peters left off – is gently empowering me to see how foolish this is. We're old. Clinging to the memory of what we used to do as runners prevents us from focusing intelligently on what we might do in future.

So what should I be doing?

Step one, suggests Pete, is to water the whole garden. In other words, try to get some speed back. Don't apathetically accept the myth that 'old runners are slow', but focus intelligently, in a targeted way, on becoming as fast as you can. (This, of course, is just what Jo Pavey advised, although I hadn't got round to doing much about it.)

Pete is a great advocate of 5,000m as the perfect target distance for the all-round runner: 'The 5k uses probably more muscle fibres at endurance level than any other race. That's why I love it.' The point isn't that it is necessarily a 'better' distance to compete at. It's just that, if you want to build a high-functioning runner's body, without significant deficits in speed, mobility, stamina or resilience, 5,000m is a great distance to train for. And that basic building work will stand you in good stead for most distances, especially within the range from 1500m to half-marathon.

The programmes Pete recommends tend to involve twelve-week cycles, in which speed work and recovery play a significant part. To over-simplify heavily: a typical week for a good 5k runner might involve one tempo session (either a single run or a series of repetitions at a comfortably hard pace that you could theoretically just about sustain for an hour); one VO_2 max session (faster intervals in which the reps are done at your current maximum 5,000m pace); one session of hill sprints or hill strides; a couple of distance runs (which between them might account for half your weekly mileage); and one or two days marked as 'OFF', in which you can, if you choose, do some form of cross-training or very easy running for aerobic purposes, but whose main purpose is recovery.

There are as many possible programmes as there are runners, and of course, the older you are, the more 'OFF' days there will be. But *all* Pete's programmes include speed work. It doesn't matter what your ultimate target is. If you want to thrive as a runner in later life, you mustn't give up on speed. Slow old runners become slow ex-runners. But old runners who work on becoming a little less slow will – if they work in a smart way – gradually rediscover a relatively full range of running motion. This approach allows us to 'recruit' more nerves, to slow down the loss of fast-twitch fibres, to build back intermediate fibres, to restore some lost elasticity and bounce to our tendons, and to get back a bit of stride length. One likely result is a dramatic improvement in race times. But the knock-on benefit is that the whole system gets trained and, over time, becomes stronger as well as faster; and stronger means better able to train.

One thing still bothers me, though: the chances of my following and sticking to a detailed, day-by-day running programme are minimal. Programmes and me don't mix. I just do what I can, when my life permits. And while I'd like to be the best runner I can be, all I really care about is continuing to be able to run, impressively or not, for pleasure and well-being. Is that really out of the question?

'Generally,' says Pete, more sympathetically than you might expect, 'I'm in favour of anything that helps people to keep running. So if the approach you've been taking works for you, more power to you. But expect to be injured. You'll slide faster. You'll keep getting slower. And if you then build up and throw in harder workouts without a plan, you'll be injured in two months. There are no shortcuts. You have to have a plan, and you have to follow it.'

I sense an unwelcome paradox closing in on me. If I want to continue to enjoy running as a casual, instinctive, spontaneous pastime, I need to take a more systematic and analytical approach. Pete agrees – and there's something about his persona that makes me value his approval very much. Late-life runners who thrive, he suggests, tend to be quite thoughtful about what they do. 'The correct training can make a huge, huge difference,' he says encouragingly. 'As long as you're not in too much of a hurry.'

But I am (I reply silently). Late life has been passing me by, and my patience is more or less spent. I want to start seizing some moments of my own.

18

Having a go

On a humid Wednesday evening towards the end of the summer, I went to Wimbledon Park athletics track to test myself in the Veterans Athletic Club 10,000m Championships.

I had hesitated long and hard before entering. I had barely even jogged 10 kilometres in recent months, and I certainly hadn't been building up to the event by patiently working through a training programme. As for racing: I hadn't raced on a track since I was a teenager. I'm just a runner, not an athlete. But it was a chance to have a go at something, and I seemed, temporarily, to be more or less injury-free. If I didn't have a go now, then when?

I wasn't much looking forward to it, though, and the days leading up to the event were shadowed with absurd dread. I've done hundreds of races in my time, but always on roads, trails or fells, where you can plod home many minutes behind the winners without anyone really noticing. In a stadium, everyone can watch you bringing up the rear, for lap after excruciating lap; and in this particular event my ordeal would be witnessed by proper competitive distance runners – real Masters athletes – who might struggle to maintain their patience if I made them wait too long.

'You mustn't say that,' said Steve Peters when I mentioned this to him. 'That's mentally damaging. You *are* a proper Masters athlete.' In theory, he was right. I was in my early sixties. I had just signed up to a Masters club, Midland Masters AC. I was about to participate in a biggish event in the Masters calendar. If that didn't make me a Masters athlete, what would? Yet I felt as anxious as a first-time jogger who shrinks from joining a parkrun for fear that 'everyone will laugh.'

On the day itself, pre-race worry almost overwhelmed me. What if I couldn't finish, or had to be timed out? What if my half-healed buttock let me down? What if I threw up? With hindsight, this seems pathetic. It was only a bloody race: no one would care what I did. But that's what happens when age gets you in its grip: your confidence goes – even when you've been a runner for decades. The thought of all that pain and despair made me sick to my stomach.

Yet neither could I quite bring myself to pull out. Competitive events for non-elite runners were still rare back then, as coronavirus waves came and went. If I didn't seize this moment, it might be months before another came along. And if I waited until I was properly fit, I might still be watching enviously from the sidelines in a decade's time, still sadly wondering what it was that enabled 'real' Masters – this strange, ostensibly fortunate minority of active late-life runners – to muddle through their physical frailties, while I could not.

So I pulled myself together. After all, how humiliating is it, really, to finish a distant last in a race? There are getting on for two million men in the UK who are, like me, in the M60–64 age category, and all but a handful of them would definitely not be making fools of themselves that evening in the VAC 10,000m championships – for the simple reason that they hadn't entered. None would come last, or strain the politeness of better athletes, or risk being laughed at by onlookers. Yet what was so admirable about that? Anyone can *not* have a go. But runners, even slow ones, are better than that.

I was still weighed down with dread when I reached Wimbledon Park, but everyone at the track seemed friendly and normal, and I wasn't quite the only person who wasn't wearing proper track shoes. The fifty competitors were spread between three races – slow, medium and fast – based on our predicted times. I was in the first, slowest race, along with four other M60s, an M55, a couple of W50s and eight others, mostly men, aged between their late sixties and their mid-seventies.

I was disappointed by the lack of W80s: I'd been hoping I might be able to sneak in front of one or two of them. On the other hand, it felt surprisingly unintimidating: just a bunch of ordinary people, getting together for some shared recreation, with minimal fuss. There was no pressure to prove anything. In any case, I told myself, perhaps someone else might feel grateful to have a slower runner in the race, to fill the last place that would otherwise have been theirs.

'All the best people are in the first race,' said Bill O'Connor, a cheerful, semi-retired, seventy-six-year-old teacher from Queen's Park, as we lined up at the start. And I realised in the last still moments before the gun went that I felt unexpectedly at home.

A crowd of seven or eight darted off in front of me at what seemed like a sensible pace. Within half a lap I was struggling – and worrying again. I couldn't possibly keep this up. All those feelings I'd been dreading surged up in my stomach: nausea, desperation, despair. Another twenty-four laps of this would be intolerable. Then I thought: 'Oh, well. Whatever.' It was too late for worrying.

So I plugged on at my own pace, wondering occasionally about the runners behind – presumably another seven or eight – who for all I knew were gathering themselves to overtake. From time to time I attempted calculations about my pace and eventual time, based on the trackside clock. But my mental arithmetic always goes to pieces when I'm racing. My provisional aim had been to get inside the W80 world record, which I vaguely remembered as just under 52 minutes, but I kept changing my mind about whether I was on schedule or not. After three or four laps I decided that I must be way behind and wondered if I should be aiming instead for the previous W80 record. I couldn't remember what that was either – 55 something? – but I had seen memorable footage of Denise LeClerc setting it, in the middle of a tropical storm in Porto Alegre, Brazil, in 2013: an eighty-year-old woman in shorts and singlet, undefeated by the driving rain, splashing defiantly through the wind-lashed puddles while young officials in knee-length macs scurried for shelter. Surely I must be able to manage something comparable, on a balmy evening in Wimbledon?

I made an effort to smile, which often helps but which I often forget to do. Within another lap, the pressure had eased. I stopped thinking about targets and comparisons and began instead to live in the moment. I thought about the simple fact that I was here, running in the melting light of a September evening; and the fact that, for the next 45 minutes or so, I could without guilt empty my mind of all thoughts apart from the need to keep putting one foot in front of the other. This was the opposite of multi-tasking modern normality. There were no interruptions, no distractions, no notifications: just running around in circles.

Every now and then I thought about upping the pace, or reproached myself for easing off. Mostly I thought how lucky I was to be among a group of strangers who, from the simple fact that they had chosen to spend their evening doing this, could be assumed to have quite a lot in common with me. I thought about the flow of my breath; about keeping up a rhythm; about going round in circles; and about the rhythms I could hear around me, of breathing and of footsteps. And I realised the strangely collective nature of what we were doing. We were rivals, but we were also equals, all in it together in the linked struggles of racing and being old.

The day's sticky heat eased as evening fell. I could no longer hear the squabbling of ducks on the nearby lake, and the squeals of ball-chasing children in the park had ebbed to a gentle babble. Squirrels emerged from the *Leylandii* and poplars bordering the stadium and played on the shadowed grass by the track. One of them scampered into the lane next to mine and ran alongside me, overtaking me on the bend. This felt unnecessarily disrespectful, but I refused to be deflated. Instead, I just kept on running.

Every now and then, someone would get lapped. Once or twice, it was me. But sometimes, too, I found myself stepping out to overtake an older straggler. It didn't take me long to get confused. Had that man overtaken me once already? And what about him – didn't I pass him at around this spot a couple of laps ago? The confusion was rather soothing, however, adding to my sense that this was a shared experience. I didn't dare run slower, or everyone would stream past me. Nor could I risk running faster, for fear that my buttock (or my stomach) might give way. With a bit of luck, however, I could be the lapper slightly more often than the lapped and, as a result, wouldn't be last to finish. That would be good enough for me.

Round and round the flat track we went, again and again, each on our own sweaty pilgrimage of twenty-five identical laps: sixteen age-battered bodies, minimally clothed, in various states of disrepair and race-induced exhaustion. Half the indignities of later life were on display, if your eyesight was good enough: thinning, thinned or absent hair; papery skin; flabby bits, skinny bits, wobbly bits; scars, bulges, blotches, tufty eyebrows, wonky teeth, curiously asymmetric muscles. There were smells, too, at times. Our ungainlier mannerisms – limps, stoops, grimaces, grunts – became more pronounced as the race went on. So did our differences in age and ability. Yet that merely emphasised the thing that united us: we were runners, running; putting on a brave face without hiding our limitations; going round in circles. That's one of the beauties of this sport: its unfiltered nakedness. You can neither hide nor pretend. All you can do is be yourself and do your best. And recognising that – in any field of life – brings both peace and strength.

Perhaps I experienced more discomfort than I now remember, but somehow, in any case, the sense that this was a shared ordeal made it feel manageable. Arthur

Schopenhauer – who spent three miserable months being educated in Wimbledon as a fifteen-year-old – might have found a moral in that. In his 1851 collection, *Studies in Pessimism*, the German philosopher argued that anyone who faced up fully to the world's suffering would immediately feel a new bond of sympathy for their fellow humans, and that the appropriate form of address between strangers should not be 'Sir' or 'Madam' but 'My fellow sufferer'. Perhaps 'suffering' was too strong a word for the varying degrees of pain we runners were experiencing, but Schopenhauer was right about the sympathy. It was impossible not to feel goodwill towards everyone on the track, even as we strove to overtake one another.

Meanwhile, strange musings came into my head, as often happens when I run. (Does any other sport offer this benefit?) I was trying to calculate what proportion of the race remained, and how much was behind me. Then it occurred to me – rather neatly, I thought – that a long race could be visualised as a metaphor for a long human life. If I was going to live to a hundred, say, then I could imagine each 100m of this 10,000m as the equivalent of a single year, with the finishing line representing my 100th birthday. It's a fairly pointless comparison, yet in terms of subjective experience it seemed astonishingly accurate. The first lap, for example, would have represented my first four years. No wonder it seemed to go on for ever: life does, at that age. And then – well, the rest is obvious. Laps two to five, notionally taking me through my childhood and my teens, also seemed to pass so slowly that it wasn't really possible to see beyond them. Yet even then, imperceptibly, I was settling into a rhythm.

Then, on laps seven, eight and nine – taking me

metaphorically into my mid-thirties – I began to feel a sense of progress. I still couldn't really imagine that point in the distant future when the race would actually be over, but a big chunk of it was now behind me, and I seemed to be getting somewhere. And then, as the shadows lengthened, I realised that the laps were passing slightly faster. I don't think I was running faster, but time, as experienced by me, had speeded up. This, of course, exactly parallels what happens in life. The sum of your lived experience grows and grows, and each new hour represents a smaller proportion of it.

Approaching the end of my fourteenth lap, I realised that I was already – metaphorically – in my mid-fifties. That's good, I thought. I'm more than halfway through. I always prefer the second half of a race. And, indeed, the fifteenth lap felt less of a struggle than any that had gone before.

Then, starting the sixteenth, I thought: that's the equivalent of my sixtieth birthday just gone. By the time I'd finished the next bend, it was like being sixty-one: the equivalent of my actual age. I seemed to be on autopilot now, but cruising quite fast. Just another lap and a bit and the race would be two-thirds done.

It still wasn't easy. My lungs strained to find enough oxygen from the unfamiliar London air, and my legs, especially my right leg, ached more with each lap. But neither was it wholly unpleasant. I was happy to be here, out in the action; happy to have showed up. And now that the finish was as good as in sight – or, at least, a single-figure number of laps away – I wasn't quite so bothered by dread of the pain to come.

In my musings, however, there was a drawback. That

mental image of the race as a symbol of my life had developed a momentum of its own. My notional sixties went past in three barely noticed laps: sixty, sixty-four, sixty-eight. Two hundred metres later I was imagining myself in my seventies. Was this the kind of blur in which my own future would pass?

Time accelerates as you age for several reasons. For a six-year-old, one year represents a sixth of everything they have ever experienced. For a sixty-year-old, it's a mere sixtieth, and so each unit of time seems briefer. The young may also experience more sensory input per hour at a literal, biological level, since neural decay makes older people receive, in effect, fewer 'frames per second'. But six-year-olds' main advantage in this respect is that, most days, they experience things that are completely novel and, as a result, vivid and intense. The moments are too full to drift by unnoticed. But how many sixty-year-olds can say the same? Perhaps that's why so many late-life athletes seem to feel an almost religious devotion to their sport: it's their lifeline to the kind of intensely lived moments that often vanish, after a certain age, from less active lives.

I was running faster by now, and the resulting discomfort made it hard to think clearly. On the bright side, however, this also distracted me from a ghastly suspicion: that, beyond the track, the remainder of my life might be stuck on fast-forward.

Still the laps slipped past, and the notional 'years' with them. Seventy-two, seventy-six: I barely noticed. Eighty, eighty-four ... It would all be over soon. There were obvious reasons for welcoming this, yet the thought also chilled me, as I realised with horrible clarity just how little of my actual life was left to me. Even as I ran, it was slipping away, and even if I survived another fifty years, each remaining year would pass faster than the one before, until, really quite soon, the final moments of my life vanished with a high-speed gurgle down the plughole.

I remembered something that Jiří Soukup once said, justifying his octogenarian passion for athletic striving: 'Life is like water. We want to hold it in our hands, but it flows through our fingers. That's why we ball our hands into fists – so that it won't flow so quickly.'

Of course! That was what I needed: fighting spirit. It was time to rage against the dying of the light. I set my sights on the runner ahead, halfway down the back straight, and accelerated with grim determination. It worked beautifully. I didn't catch him – at least, not on this lap – but by the time I accepted the need to ease off a little my perception of time had been transformed. Each minute felt like an hour, and the idea of continuing like this for another three-and-a-half laps seemed absurd. Then, after an easier spell, the remaining distance began to seem manageable again, so I dialled up the effort again to an unsustainable level, then eased off, then surged again . . . and time barely seemed to be passing at all.

I crossed the line neck-and-neck with the winner, Steve Oliver, a whippet-thin M60 from Winchester. Two laps later, the bell sounded for my own last lap. By then I had put in so many bursts of extra effort that I wasn't even sure I could keep going for a whole 400m. Yet when I focused on my lifespan analogy the remaining distance seemed too short. *I'm not ready to die*, I kept saying to myself. *I haven't finished.* I still have more inside me, more to give . . .

I threw every scrap of my remaining strength at the problem, and I think I may have overtaken three people on the final 200m, screaming to myself internally 'I DON'T WANT TO DIE YET!' I finished in a glorious cloud of pain, five-and-a-half minutes behind Oliver – who was already looking absurdly fresh while I lurched for the rails by the stand. I leaned on them for what may have been five minutes, gasping for breath. A nearby paramedic gave a reassuring smile. She could tell that the only thing I was in danger of dying from was happiness.

The gentle beauty of the aftermath more than justified the agonies of the race, and the anxious gloom before-hand. We lingered near the finish until we had clapped the last runner home. Then we lingered some more. Perhaps this wasn't sensible, as our bodies cooled, but why break the spell? We congratulated one another, with words and gestures. We chatted vaguely about how it had been for us. We enthused about how nice it was to have had a proper race organised for us, after all those empty months. And, paradoxically, we enthused about how particularly great it felt, now that it was over.

I can't tell you who said what to whom. Different con-versations have blurred and merged in my memory, just as the scents of our evaporating sweat – a dozen or more distinctive odours – mingled in the evening air. But I do remember a long chat with Joe Aspinall, a pale-as-death eighty-three-year-old who told me with pride that he was 'eight and a half stone of skin and bone' and that he had 'never been to a gym in my life'. This hardly needed say-ing, but his frail appearance was deceptive. He has been running for over fifty years, including more than thirty as a member of Veterans Athletic Club, and you won't find many VAC events where he isn't racing. This one was a rare exception. He was still recovering from a fall on the finishing line the previous week and was limiting himself this evening to handing out drinks; but he would, he assured me, be back racing the following week. Caution, he explained, was the secret of his resilience. 'If you look after your body, your body will look after you. I'm not sixty any more. I've had to slow down. Top athletes take so much out of their bodies, but I just do what I can.'

What he doesn't do, he added, is sit at home doing nothing. 'I never stop. I'm not one to sit indoors – I get agitated.' When he isn't running, he's hill-walking; getting around London, where he lives, he walks everywhere: 'The more stairs, the better.' He has no interest in scientific training. He just walks a lot and runs a little. 'I can still do what I did forty years ago. I just I don't do as much of it.'

I also remember resuming my pre-race conversation with Bill O'Connor, whose jolly, bearded face looked distinctly haggard when he crossed the line. He had, he confessed, found the race a bit of a struggle. His arthritic left knee had been playing up, as it sometimes does – possibly, he explained, as a result of years of slightly lop-sided running. 'Years ago I slipped and fell in the Watford half-marathon, and it turned out that I'd damaged a nerve, permanently. I didn't believe it at first, but two different specialists told me.' So he carried on with the nerves he had left, and was doing pretty well until, five years ago, he was attacked and almost killed by a dog while he was out on a training run. 'I knew I had to get to a hospital really, really quickly,' he said, spelling out the details with cheerful relish. But he lived to tell the tale and, once again, he coaxed his battered body back into regular running. He still runs with a heavily bandaged right arm, though, which isn't conducive to perfect balance, and I don't suppose it helps that he's built more like a rugby player – or a bear – than a distance runner.

But who needs perfection, when you have a runner's heart? Like his friend Ken Jones, Bill O'Connor is one of the handful of 'Ever-Presents' who have never missed a London Marathon. His forty-first was, at this point, only three weeks away. This evening's race, he explained, was just part of his marathon preparations and, while it could have gone better, 'I came through in one piece. That's all I care about.'

Much later, I was amazed to discover that I'd come third in the race (and even when the faster races had been run I was fifth out of eight M60s). My time was about 5 minutes quicker than I had at one point feared, although I'm too embarrassed to share it here. Let's just say that it was couple of minutes outside the world record for a seventy-year-old woman – and 13 or 14 minutes slower than I might have hoped for, with that much effort, thirty years ago. But so what?

The simple fact that continued to fill me with absurd happiness was that, like Bill O'Connor, I had come through in one piece. I was back competing again, being a runner, an athlete even. I had run 10,000m, not fast or well but without consciously slacking at any point. I had had a new and interesting experience. And, putting an upbeat spin on it, I hadn't come last in my age group at the big(-gish) annual championship of one of the world's most prestigious veterans' athletics clubs. It wasn't much. But it was a start.

More sobering was the thought of how intimidated I had felt beforehand. I'm a hardened competitor, by most standards, with decades of off-track racing behind me, yet I hadn't felt confident at all about self-identifying as a Masters athlete in a stadium event, because – well, because I'm no longer the man I used to be. And if that's how it felt to me, imagine how it might seem to a novice, toying with the idea of having a go at running in later life. No wonder Masters athletics is a niche pursuit.

So I made a resolution. From now on, I will stop thinking of myself as an old man or a has-been. I will think of myself instead as an athlete: not a good one, but an athlete none the less, with motives that include the continuing possibility of improvement. Above all, I will be shameless. I will turn up where and when I feel like it, and run as well as I can, until I can run no more (after which, like Amby Burfoot, I will walk). And if people don't like it, they can look away.

By the time these thoughts occurred to me, I was getting cold and stiff. So I said goodbye to my fellow-lingerers and trudged across the park to my car, enjoying the last of the sun's rays on my sweat-sticky back and noting with pleasure that my hamstring was nagging less now than it had before the race. Maybe I did have a future as a runner – if I didn't get carried away.

At the car park, I felt an uncharacteristic twinge of embarrassment at the state of my grubby, battered, ancient Nissan Micra. It seemed to be lowering the tone, compared with the shiny new vehicles around it. Then I thought: oh well, it works for me; and in any case it's all I've got.

And that, I realised driving home, was essentially the

big lesson I needed to take from my evening's experiences. Frailty is a fact of later life, for runners as for everyone else. We will never be wholly undamaged again, physically or, for that matter, emotionally; but these battered versions of ourselves are what we have to work with for the rest of our lives. This means that, like Joe Aspinall, we should manage our bodies with care, like the worn-out, unreliable machines they are; but also that, like Bill O'Connor, we shouldn't be afraid to use them. Running in later life is about survival. But it is also about running – even at the occasional risk of running ourselves into the ground.

19

Time and motion

'Is it age?' says Nigel Crompton. 'Or is it time? I don't know. People accumulate things.'

I can see what he means. I've spent the last fifteen minutes rattling through the edited highlights of my life's injury history. Nigel told me to include everything, but there really isn't time. In any case, how could I remember? So I mention a selection of the uglier mishaps: the time I impaled my foot on a rusty spike in the mid-1970s; the torn left ankle ligaments, from a 1984 game of football, that have never quite been right since; the suitcase-lifting misjudgement in 1990 that still hurts today; the worst of my many fell-running sprains (right ankle this time) in 1992; and so on, all the way up to the torn calf in 2014, and the hernia in 2015, and beyond. Up to a dozen fairly hard-core ankle sprains have blurred together: who knows or cares which was right and which was left, or when they happened? And that's before we start on the secondary injuries: the iliotibial band syndrome, the Achilles tendi-nitis, the alternating knee pains, the sore hamstrings, and so on, all of which presumably began, once, with an actual trauma somewhere. Major omissions are still popping into my head days later: the torn bicep (still misshapen twenty years later), the impinged shoulder, the impaled hand, the motorcycle crash, the toes misshapen from ill-fitting shoes in childhood . . .

The odd thing is, this litany of damage is just the wear-and-tear from a pretty average baby-boomer life. I think I must be clumsier than average, and I'm childishly bad at waiting for injuries to heal properly. But I'm hardly a daredevil action man. I've just spent a longish time being alive.

Yet it turns out that all these actively acquired traumas are only part of my full tally of damage. Nigel also wants to know about my lifestyle history, my occupational history, how much time I spend driving, what position I adopt when working at my computer: anything that might have affected my body in the periods between bouts of action. I don't know him well enough to share my (mercifully limited) history of emotional hurt, although some therapists would argue that this was relevant too. But I've already given him plenty of raw material to work with.

The point, he explains, is that most runners' injuries aren't running injuries at all. 'The people I treat come to me with lifestyle issues, occupational issues, or a history of traumatic injury.' He cites a range of examples: the van driver who sits in a van all day and on a sofa all evening, and has hips that are tilted forward; the person who has spent twenty years at a desk, always bending to the left to pick up heavy files; the lifelong golfer whose pelvis is rotated off-centre; the boxer twisted at the shoulder; or the woman who spent months on crutches from a skiing accident decades ago, whose posture has shifted to compensate. 'The body adapts to whatever it thinks we want it to do. But when we run, running finds these adaptations out.' To call them running injuries misses the point. 'It is the baggage that we bring to running.'

Nigel is a former NHS nurse who found an unexpected calling as a running therapist in middle age. Previously, he had run only for general fitness, to help with his hobby of Chinese martial arts. Then, in his forties, he got more serious. He joined a running club. He started trying to understand what the sport involved, did a coaching qual-ification, became a fell-runner, and completed some fairly hard-core off-road races, including the Marathon des Sables. In 2015 he took redundancy from the NHS and opened a small high street shop near his home in the Wirral.

He called it the Runners' Hub, and used it, initially, to sell running kit. But runners love expertise almost as much as we love shiny new products, and in due course the little shop, staffed by local enthusiasts, became one of those places where people go not just to buy stuff but to talk about what's going on in their sport: gossip, prod-ucts, gimmicks; the best new training tips and – of course – what to do about their injuries. For the shop's first year, Nigel had been struggling with his own injury: a painful psoas muscle that he was initially advised to treat, in the conventional way, by stretching. The treat-ment worked for a while, but the problem kept coming back. It took him several years to realise that, in fact, the stretching was making it worse.

The problem started, he believes, with an ankle sprain in the Carneddau mountains in north Wales, exacer-bated by a five-mile hobble back to civilisation. That seemed to heal, but an instinct to protect the injured joint had embedded itself in his gait. 'I hiked up my hip to keep off it, so this' – he points to the psoas – 'is being held long, and that compensatory mechanism is what leads to the problem. So the psoas is being held taut, like a tired old piece of elastic, and the last thing I need is to stretch it. What I actually need is to strengthen it.'

By the time he had worked that out, he had worked out quite a few other things. He had heard endless stories about persistent injuries, from his running friends, from the runners who passed through his shop and from the runners he met through coaching. And now he had his own frustratingly wide experience of conventional treatments. He could see that each method he tried had something to offer, from mainstream physiotherapy to podiatry, osteopathy and chiropractic. But he also felt that they were missing something.

He resolved to learn more about biomechanics. He qualified as a corrective exercise specialist with the National Association of Sports Medicine. And in recent years he has had a little basement treatment room beneath the shop, in which he is currently giving my battered body a quick once-over. But most of what he is telling me reflects his encounters with a succession of therapists – Joe Kelly in Devon, Simon Jones in north Wales – from the influential Anatomy in Motion (AIM) school of therapeutic thought. For AIM practitioners, physiology means little without motion. The body is a highly evolved organism for movement, and persistent movement-associated pain is likely to reflect acquired distortions of natural movement patterns. Healing, in this model, comes from re-learning natural movement patterns; or, rather, from helping the body to re-learn those patterns. The method was created by the London-based therapist Gary

Ward, who based it on what he called the Flow Motion Model: a detailed, three-dimensional map of the positioning of 207 bones and 360 joints at every stage in the gait cycle. This shows, among other things, how interdependent the various parts of the body are, and how the relationships between them change as the body moves. Ward has described his approach in a successful book, *What the Foot?*, and many runners have found it spectacularly effective. Others, including me, have found it helpful for broadening our focus. It's easy to develop tunnel vision with injuries: you focus on a specific symptom, and, the longer it continues, the more that dominates your perceptions. Thinking in terms of a whole-body system of natural movement empowers us to notice issues that may be closer to the heart of the problem, and to see healing less as a distant, unattainable goal and more as simple reset.

'I see this all the time,' says Nigel. 'People come to me with injuries that won't go away. And they've had it looked at – let's say it's the knee – and from then on that's the only thing anyone looks at. Therapists focus on one thing. But I won't do that. I do a whole-body assessment. I take an occupational history, I take injuries, lifestyle things . . .' As for healing, it's not so much treatment as re-education. 'You're actually teaching your body: "This is what I need to do . . ."'

In my case, he has spotted a number of problems. A foot-pressure gauge reveals that my centre of mass in gait isn't going through my feet in the right places, especially in the left foot. ('You can live with that on the right, but here, that's not good . . .') There is visible instability in the metatarsophalangeal (MTP) joint. And a simple knee-to-the-wall test shows that – probably as a result of all those fell-running sprains – I have almost completely lost my ability to dorsiflex (i.e. bend the ankle so that the shin approaches the toes), on both sides. 'I've never had someone score this badly before,' says Nigel, with a hint of awe in his voice.

One effect of these malfunctions is that my feet – especially the left – can no longer pronate properly. 'So you're having to compensate, because the foot's not engaging properly. And because it's unstable, the joints above it are trying to control it.' All of which suggests that, if my running is causing me persistent pains that migrate seemingly at random between knees, hamstrings and pelvis, that's hardly surprising.

On the bright side, there's a plausible route to recovery: all I need is for my feet to re-learn the art of natural articulation. In other words – in Gary Ward's phrase – to 'teach the body to recognise normal'.

Nigel gives me a programme of 'mobility homework' to help me do this. It includes half a dozen movements or movement chains to be repeated until they become instinctive again. 'Don't think of them as exercises,' says Nigel. 'Think of them as movements. Make them fluid.' The aim isn't to strengthen anything, or even to stretch anything. In fact, the movements don't *achieve* anything at all. They are the end, not the means: basic building blocks of natural human motion, which the buffetings of life have caused my body to forget, but which could, with a little practice, be relearnt.

The homework includes a series of turning movements through which my foot can learn – helped, initially, by a small wedge – what proper, natural pronation feels like:

'so the foot splats on the ground like a cowpat'. Another movement chain seems to involve pretending to be a spectacularly flamboyant waiter: front leg bent obsequiously, back leg straight, opposite arm stretched forward at the front as if with a proffered tray (to encourage thoracic rotation), other arm curled sideways over the head as if it had just whipped a silver cover off a flambéed steak (to encourage lateral flexion of the spine).

I feel as though I am being given a lot to remember: pushing off evenly through my first and fifth MTP joints ('your met-heads'); landing on the inter-ossial area ('just below where the laces are tied'); and so on. But this isn't about conscious learning. 'There's no point telling somebody, "You should do it like this," because every footstep takes about a fifth of a second.' If my body re-familiarises itself with the sensations of natural movement, however, it will instinctively do what needs to be done. 'A lot of this is about neuromuscular pathways. It'll happen over time. Just keep doing it until it flows.'

It helps that Nigel is good at giving simple little concepts to keep in mind: splatting the foot like a cowpat; imagining my footfalls as landings ('If we jumped off a step, we would land naturally just here'); not clenching my toes ('Keep asking yourself: "Are my toes relaxed? Are my toes relaxed?"'). He often advises people to imagine themselves running without arms and legs. 'How would you achieve forward motion, if you were running on stumps?' The answer, you quickly work out, is that you would use rotation, of the lumbar spine at the bottom and the thoracic spine at the top. 'Power comes from the spine,' he says, and directs me to Serge Gracovetsky's groundbreaking book, *The Spinal Engine*, for a physiological explanation. In fact, the point is obvious, once you think about it, and is clearly visible in the running of, for example, Eliud Kipchoge. But if all your attention is focused on what's happening in your legs, the chances are you won't think about it.

The big benefit of the 'stumps' idea for me is not that it helps me generate power but that it helps me move more freely. When I run with my spine, my body starts to shed its acquired inhibitions. That's part of the point. 'When I see runners who aren't happy running,' says Nigel, 'the movement is really compromised. Everything is smaller, shorter. There's no extension, there's no rotation, there's no movement. I try to get them to learn the connectivity between various bits. It's not about understanding anatomy. It's about body awareness.'

Is it realistic, I ask, for me to hope to get back to perfect posture and gait after so many years of habitual distortion? He looks me up and down and sucks his teeth. 'Perfect? Possibly not. But I think we can get to an optimum.'

Much of his teaching is done in workshops. Local runners sign up in small groups for a six-week programme, and 'all these little things about connectivity are just built up week by week.' The workshops include a lot of jumping – which he demonstrates with a series of seemingly effortless leaps in which his feet come about four foot off the floor. This not only strengthens the legs but 'teaches them what they need to do': not just powering off but landing naturally. 'Jumping is running,' he adds, 'and running is jumping.'

The workshops also include a lot of one-legged work – which Nigel demonstrates with a series of seemingly effortless one-legged squats. 'Running is a one-legged sport,' he says. 'By definition, when you run, you're either on one leg or the other.' But both legs need to be fully functional, or imbalances develop and grow: 'The stronger leg does more of the work, so the stronger leg keeps getting stronger, and over time the imbalance just gets more and more and more.' Doing one-legged exercises, however, 'people quickly find out if they have a problem' and, over time, learn to re-balance.

Some find the work harder than others. 'I had an email from a guy who was seventy years of age, and he only took up running during the lockdown. Would my workshops be suited to him? So I thought, yes, but I'll have to do lots of regressions of exercises to make them really easy. But he was probably the most athletic person in that room. He had body awareness.'

Developing awareness, by which he means a sense of when the body is moving as nature intended and when it isn't, is, he believes, the essential first step in any runner's journey towards full mobility, which itself is essential to injury-free running. 'You can tell somebody to change their running form: to run with higher cadence, to land more mid-foot, to run upright, to lean – whatever. If there aren't good movement patterns in place, these changes are like building a house without a foundation.' But once you can distinguish between the different sensations of 'natural' and 'unnatural', you will instinctively begin to feel your way back towards natural movements and, in due course, full mobility.

Mobility, he adds, should not be confused with flexibility. 'Put your hand flat on the table, palm down, and see how far you can raise your middle finger. That's mobility.

Now see how far you can lift your middle finger if you pull it with your other hand. That's flexibility.' Flexibility is useful for contortionists, and perhaps also for gymnasts and ballet dancers. Runners just need a full range of motion.

Nigel recently published a book making this very point. *My Border Collie Doesn't Stretch* charts his journey from chronically injured runner to qualified, injury-free therapist, while emphasising his growing disillusionment with static stretching (the kind that runners of my generation have traditionally been urged to do before and after each run). The book is short and very readable, but its distinctiveness lies not so much in the anti-stretching message – which some modern runners might consider uncontroversial – as in its use of Mollie, Nigel's dog, as a positive role model. All mammals prepare themselves before vigorous activity, he argues, but only humans do so by attempting with great discomfort to lengthen their muscles and tendons. What other creatures do – and we have all seen cats and dogs doing it – is awaken their neuromuscular pathways by taking their bodies through a full range of motion. The technical term for this is 'pandiculation', but it's basically the entirely instinctive (and comfortable) kind of movement that you might observe when a toddler yawns extravagantly on waking up. It's also the kind of movement that Nigel is teaching me through what I still think of as his remedial exercises. But they're not exercises: they're awakenings, making sure that the lines of communication are fully open so that the body can move fully and freely.

Nigel advises me to think of my 'homework' not just as a remedial routine but as a valuable part of my pre-run warm-up. 'A lot of these movements are about making a neuromuscular connection,' he says. 'That's why that compound exercise I showed you is so good. Do it before you run, and you take it into the run with you.' As he says this, he demonstrates again the movement that I think of as the 'flamboyant waiter' routine; and, as usual, he makes it seem fluid, controlled and effortless. It occurs to me that Nigel is actually quite an athlete.

You wouldn't pick him out as a tough guy, with his modest manner, his big glasses, his short, greying beard, and his thoughtful, slightly worried-looking face. But he is in astonishingly good shape, perfectly balanced and with unrestricted mobility; and, it seems, still improving as a runner. 'I'm actually in a lot better shape now than I was at fifty. I'm certainly a lot more mobile.' He's also eagerly plotting his next hard-core off-road challenge (the Bob Graham Round) and checking out target times for various distances for next time he moves up an age category.

'Sometimes,' he says, 'I do regret not having learnt all this when I was twenty. Because then you think, "Oh, what could I have done?" But actually I quite enjoy the sense of getting older. I like being able to talk to the young runners in my shop, and then to tell them: I'm a sixty-year-old runner who never, ever stretches, yet I've got full mobility. And I'm not the only one,' he adds. 'Some of the old guys you see on the fells, they just go on and on for ever.'

I wish I was feeling similarly indestructible, but first I need to get down to some serious homework. Already, however, I am starting to see a path ahead. For too long, I realise, I have been thinking in terms of forcing my body to do things against its will. Whether it's stretching or remedial physio, weightlifting or speed drills, my whole emotional approach has tended to involve using sheer willpower to force my body into shape. No pain, no gain: that's what we were taught. Yet maybe what I need most, at this stage of life, is to relax a bit more: to let go of all those accumulated knots of caution and self-protection, and trust my body to do what it does naturally.

When I leave the Runners' Hub and walk back to my car, I seem to be almost hyper-aware of my movements. Are my toes relaxed? Are my feet articulating? Are they hip-width apart? Am I putting pressure through my met-heads? I barely notice the cold and wet of the darkening December afternoon. Move freely, I tell myself. Let yourself out of 'protect state'. Think balance. Think mobility.

I feel strangely alive, and unusually full of hope. It may not be quick, shedding the accumulated physical baggage of a lifetime. But I think I might enjoy the attempt.

On a corner, a cluster of young people hunches against the drizzle. There's an ill-at-ease moodiness about them that reminds me of my own youth. One is drinking from a can; another is eating a pungent take-away. No one is saying much, everyone seems ill at ease, and I can discern no signs of happiness. It's strange, I reflect. They are young. They have their whole lives before them, as I did once. I ought to envy them. Yet somehow I don't.

Later, this takes me to another thought. The young can get away with almost anything. They can eat junk, stay out all night partying, lurch chaotically from one relationship to the next, and compete energetically in sport with neither restraint nor regular preparation. And they have no idea how lucky they are. But age forces us to grow up. We discover with increasing immediacy that the gifts life has given us are perishable, and finite in number. And often it sinks in, eventually, that the less we cherish them, the sooner we'll lose them.

But this is also the privilege of age. Finally, just as it is slipping away, you appreciate the value of what you have been given. And if you're very lucky, there will still be something to cherish, and time to feel thankful for it.

20

Second lives

Life always beats you in the end. Sometimes, though, you get another stab at it before you're through. Yoko Nakono was just turning seventy when things really started to go her way.

'I had a very hard life when I was young,' she told me, a few weeks before her eighty-sixth birthday. 'I lost my father when I was really young. I was the oldest child, with six siblings, so I had to look after everybody. The whole family.' She left her Tokyo school at fifteen and took a job in the local Seiko factory. She didn't enjoy it much: she had hoped for a more creative career. But 'everyone was depending on me,' so she got on with it.

Half a century later, she was still getting on with it. The factory job had eventually come to an end, and she had retrained as a dressmaker, eventually even opening a small boutique selling handmade clothes. But the balance of her life, at work and at home, remained the same. Other people's needs came first. She never got round to marriage or children, yet domestic duties dominated those parts of her existence that weren't defined by the daily grind of earning a living – especially when her mother's health deteriorated. This, it seemed, was all that life had to offer her. 'I never had any fun,' she says today, matter-of-factly.

She did, however, have one release, which was skiing: a popular and accessible recreation in Japan. When time and finances permitted, she escaped to the mountains, and over the years she became good enough to qualify as an instructor, although she never actually worked as one. Then she turned sixty. Paid work began to dry up, and skiing became unfeasibly extravagant.

Seeking a cheaper recreation, Nakano tried joining in with her younger sister when she went jogging. 'It wasn't really running,' she says now, but it wasn't difficult. The years passed, and it became a habit. She didn't take it seriously, though. There wasn't time. Her energies still went mostly into caring for her elderly mother, while to make ends meet she found part-time employment doing menial work in a care home.

Then, as she approached seventy, her sister and brother-in-law suggested that Yoko join them on a family holiday in Hawaii, and her nephew suggested that, while they were there, it might be fun to enter the famous Honolulu Marathon. Yoko, who wasn't used to doing things just for fun, decided to give it a go.

She had six months to prepare, and she used the time wisely. 'I knew from skiing that it's really important to get your basic form right.' So she went to a sports shop which offered seminars for novice runners, and signed up for a course of them. Only when she was certain that she was running as nature intended did she start to build up her mileage.

It felt a bit strange at first – 'I didn't know anyone else my age who was doing this' – and she initially felt embarrassed going outside her home in shorts. But she got used to running on a pleasant path alongside the Tama river, not far from her home in Nishikamata, south of Tokyo. The weeks passed, and the miles mounted up.

When the marathon came, 'It was rather easy.' Nakano's time, 4:44:44, was not only highly respectable for a W70 but also, to her eyes, spookily neat. 'Somehow, I felt it must be my destiny.'

She may have been right. In the fifteen years since then, running has transformed her life. She has run getting on for twenty-five marathons, including a world-record 3:53:42 in Otawara when she was seventy-six, and an equally world-beating 4:11:45 in Tokyo when she was eighty-one. For five or six years she improved continuously. (That's one of the joys of being a late starter.) Then, in her late seventies, she levelled off – in contrast to the late seventies slump that most runners experience.

She also expanded her repertoire, after discovering Japan's thriving track scene for older runners. 'I found that there were Masters competitions, and that you can do it until you're a hundred years old.' So she had a go, and she loved it. 'It brought me to many interesting places, and I met so many interesting people. When you ski you only interact with the people in your group. When you run you intermingle with lots of people you don't know. That is a great thing. Normally, I would never have met such people.'

What she's slower to mention is that, since taking to the track, she has achieved a breathtaking dominance of her age group. At the 2018 World Masters Athletics Championships in Málaga, she won four golds, at 800m, 5,000m, 10,000m and marathon; and by the end of her time as a W80 she held six outdoor world records, at 800m, 1500m, 3,000m, 5,000m, 10,000m and marathon.

It hasn't all been easy. Her hopes of a fast time in the 2013 Boston Marathon were derailed by an intestinal problem that required a major stomach operation. She still wasn't back to her best for the following year's race but ran it anyway, fell twice (waving too exuberantly to roadside friends), yet picked herself up each time to finish, bruised but unbroken, in 4:53:39. Two years later, as an eighty-year-old, she ran the same race seven-and-a-half minutes faster; but even then she was still recovering.

The following year, however, she was back to her best, as she proved in the 2017 Tokyo Marathon – her fastest for five years. 'That was my dream marathon,' she remembers. 'I ran exactly as I planned.' The resulting world record, 4:11:45, has yet to be threatened.

It also made her famous. Japan has the world's most 'super-aged' population – one woman in three is over sixty-five – and a national passion for running that takes many Westerners by surprise. So it's hardly surprising that Masters athletics is thriving there. Brett Larner, US-born editor of the acclaimed Japan Running News website, reckons that 'the World Masters record books would look very different if all the results from Japan were routinely transliterated'. Champions such as the late centenarian sprinter Hidekichi Miyazaki – the self-styled 'Golden Bolt' – have achieved national celebrity status, and a string of other late-life world-beaters could be considered household names: from Yoshihisa Hosaka (former M60 world marathon record holder) and Mariko Yugeta (the first W60 to run a sub-three-hour marathon) to nonagenarian sprinters such as Hiroo Tanaka and

Mitsu Morita or the world-record-breaking M95 distance runner Yoshimitsu Miyauchi. Nakano, too, has been part of this prestigious pantheon in recent years, which is disconcerting for someone who spent so many decades in life's background. She is thrilled, however, that people seem to find her example inspiring. 'Lots of people talk to me, and say that it's really encouraging to watch me. Sometimes they tell me: "I had been thinking of quitting running, but now I won't."'

Does Nakano have a secret? Perhaps, but she doesn't know what. There is nothing fancy about her training, beyond her focus on good biomechanics. (She has done several other courses on running form, including one with Olympic marathon runner Akio Usami.) Otherwise, she just runs, four times a week, averaging between 20 and 30 miles a week, and that's about it. She does nothing for strength ('I hate strength training') and little for flexibility ('I just stretch for five minutes before a race'), and suspects that 'the reason I don't get injured is that I don't push myself to my limits.' As for diet: 'I just eat normal food.' She does, however, do a lot of sleeping: 'I sleep really well.'

She has never had a running injury, unless you count the grazes and bruising from those falls in Boston. 'If you have correct running form you won't get injured,' she explains. Perhaps it helps, too, that she came to the sport late, sparing her joints too many years of battering. And it can't do any harm that she has a defiantly determined mindset. After that 2013 stomach operation, she started work on her recovery while still an inpatient, walking up to 7 kilometres a day in the hospital corridors.

Yet it's hard not to speculate that the core of her secret

may be something more fundamental than that: she enjoys her running. Asked for her advice for newcomers to the late-life running scene, she says: 'If you feel you are having fun you'll keep doing it, and if you have fun, you'll get faster. The most important thing is to enjoy yourself.'

In video footage of Nakano running, you notice her upright posture and her excellent balance, with small, light, neat steps. Above all, however, you notice her smile. It can hardly be easy for her: a marathon isn't easy at any age. Yet she always appears to be having fun.

She feels her age more than she used to. 'I do things slower, and my eyesight is getting worse.' She notices, too, that 'people I used to run with have either stopped running or passed away.' She has cut back her part-time job to one day a week, and she doesn't think she can afford to go to any further world championships. 'Otherwise I'll spend more on running than I did on skiing.' But she cannot imagine giving up on a sport which has given her the happiest years of her life.

'Sometimes I wonder, 'How long can I do this?' But I'm not going to stop. If I stop running, what am I going to do?'

In any case, she adds, she still has records to break. 'I want to break all the world records for eighty-five-year-olds, from 800m to marathon.' She has the target times written down in her notebook, and if you compare them with her W80 records they appear to be well within her grasp. Meanwhile, she continues to emphasise the joy her late-life adventure has brought her. She says that she loves the way it brings her into contact with other age groups – 'It is wonderful to talk to younger people' – and she loves the sense that, finally, she is fulfilling her potential. 'This is the prime of my life,' she laughs, 'and everyone else in the family is really happy for me. This is my time now.'

There is something uplifting about Nakono's modestly told story: the ordinary woman who lived an ordinary life, only to blossom when a new door opened to her in what is usually dismissed as old age. But this is a pattern that appears repeatedly in late-life running, and one of the beauties of the sport is that you never know when another new, miraculous talent is going to burst into life without warning, seemingly from nowhere. You can be pretty sure, however, that such a talent is out there some-where, waiting to be awakened.

Nakono's W80 world records seem unassailable now, but so, once, did the records she broke. Nakono was still a half-hearted jogger when the previous *grand dame* of W80 running won her first world championship gold medal, and no one could have predicted that a novice from Nishi-kamata would before long dethrone the great Denise LeClerc – except perhaps for Leclerc herself, whose own early life had, if anything, been even less promising.

LeClerc's childhood, she told me shortly before her retirement, was overshadowed by the terror of the German bombing of Paris in 1940 and by the subsequent privations of the Occupation; and, she says, by a 'serious, angry' father 'without warmth or love'. Her twenties and early thirties were then blighted by severe and recurrent health crises, including ovarian cysts, a blocked intestine and serious spinal problems. Rarely well enough to work, she had had two major operations by the time she was thirty-three, one of which she only just survived. 'The surgeon saved my life,' she recalls.

It probably didn't help that she was a smoker, but, given the state she was in, it barely seemed worth giving thought to long-term health, let alone fitness. When she did venture out into the world for the first time as a frail, skeletal, anxious thirty-something, she may have looked older, and more confident, than she was. Seeking a role in life, she trained, qualified and found employment as a beautician, travelled a lot and alone on the hippie trail, and did absolutely nothing to suggest athletic aptitude or inclination. Even when she gave up smoking, aged thirty-nine, it was only because she considered it 'incompatible with my job'.

Then, when she was in her mid-forties, a client persuaded her to try 'fitness walking'. She did, enjoyed it, and gradually drifted into race walking. She joined an athletics club when she was forty-seven, and suddenly felt, for the first time, a sense of belonging. When she first raced in the club colours, 'I was so happy I thought my heart would burst out of my chest.' Even so, for several years life's interruptions meant that her involvement in the sport was inconsistent. By the 1990s, however, she was competing internationally as a race-walker, winning one world and two European golds. Then, in 2002, after a frustrating disqualification in the 10km road walk at the world championships in Brisbane, she decided to try running. She was sixty-eight and, just like Nakano in *her* late sixties, she was about to begin the best part of her life.

Over the next few years, LeClerc began her life's most important personal relationship, with a younger journalist and Masters athlete called François Poncin. They moved to their current home in Cluny, near Dijon. She joined her current club, Athlétic Club Chenôve, which she adores ('We are all friends, young and less young, and there is no allusion to my being the oldest'). And she became the best distance runner of her age group in the world. Her peak was in 2013 and 2014, as she moved from W75 to W80. She won two European W75 golds (at 1500m and 5,000m) just a few weeks before her eightieth birthday and then, a few weeks after it, won W80 gold for the 10,000m, the 20km race-walk and the 5,000m at the world championships in Porto Alegre, Brazil. The first two were world records; the third should have been but wasn't ratified because of an administrative foul-up. Furious, LeClerc broke that record again at the following year's European championships in Izmir, Turkey ('I worked so hard that it was out of the question that I would fail to obtain the record') – by which time she also held the world record for the half-marathon and the world indoor record for 3,000m. The latter, at the French championships in Sorbonne, was her 'most beautiful' record: 'Everyone in the stands was shouting my name standing up.' The invalid of fifty years earlier had become a national sporting icon.

A hamstring injury in 2015 brought that purple patch to an end, but there were more records and medals to come. Altogether, LeClerc has been a world champion sixteen times and a European champion nineteen times, has set seven world records and, the last time I looked, was France's most medalled and celebrated veteran athlete of any age. Now eighty-nine, she exudes fitness and well-being, and if there sometimes seems to be a hint of youthful anxiety in her posture, this vanishes when she laughs or runs. The pandemic has taken the edge off her sporting hunger – 'I haven't renewed my licence as an athlete' – but nothing will alter her love of running. 'I'll always run for fitness,' she told me.

Like Nakano, LeClerc knows that she has much to be thankful for. Her two decades as a runner have, she says, 'filled me with happiness, enormous feelings, the strongest of my life'; and it seems reasonable to describe her experience of late life as enviable. Yet whether she could be said to be lucky, in the sense of having been dealt a better-than-average physiological hand at birth, is, given her back story, a moot point.

But that is another beauty of Masters athletics. It isn't just about genetic luck. Instead, for many late-starting world-beaters, there are other qualities involved: courage, determination, positivity, and a capacity – which most of us lose as we age – to get more excited about the present and the future than about the past. I've sensed this repeatedly in my dealings with Angela Copson, the UK's most successful over-sixty female distance and middle-distance runner of the past fifteen years.

Copson – currently erasing Le Clerc's W75 times from the record books and in due course likely to threaten Nakono's W80 times as well – inspires people for many reasons. She is kind, modest, high-achieving and infectiously positive, and she brims with vitality. But perhaps her most distinctive quality is her habit of enthusing about her current life, not her past.

She was born in 1947, in a smoky village pub just outside Northampton. Her early years were dominated by domestic misery and sickness. She herself was in and out of hospital, but her parents' problems troubled her most.

'My child life is not one I like to think about,' she says with a shudder.

She left home as soon as she could and found live-in employment as a sixteen-year-old stable hand at a local riding school. The physical demands almost defeated her: 'I weighed six-and-a-half-stone. I was so weak, so tired.' But there were five other young women working and living with her, and from them she learned, for the first time, 'what it was like to share a happy home'.

The six became lifelong friends. Copson learned to love horses, and grew stronger, physically and emotionally. One job led to another, involving horses and nannying. More lasting friendships resulted. Then, in her early twenties, she met a local builder, Harry Copson. They married in 1969, and only then did what she thinks of as her 'real' life begin.

Sport, however, played little part in it. She was far from sedentary, but 'everything I did was around our son and daughter.' She played badminton with them, went riding with them, messed about with them in the garden. 'I wanted for my children what I didn't have for myself, and that was a family.'

It never occurred to her to wonder about her own athletic potential, let alone to think of herself as exceptional. If anything, she was grateful for the normality of being an ordinary, busy mother. Then as now, her priorities were simple: 'Family comes first.'

But life happens to families too. The children grew up and left home. 'I was devastated. It seemed to happen so quickly.' Harry, meanwhile, grew older too. One day, on a walking holiday in Devon in 2006, he complained of chest pains that turned out to signify serious heart trouble. He was later treated at the John Radcliffe Hospital, Oxford, which fitted him out with stents and sent him home with a rigorous exercise programme.

Unfortunately, explains Copson, 'he'd completely lost his confidence really. He needed motivation.' So when he went out for his daily bike ride, she took to 'trotting along beside him'. It wasn't how either of them had imagined spending their mid-sixties: they'd been thinking more in terms of leisurely holidays. But it was 'a second chance', and they took it. Copson then decided that they needed to raise some money for the John Radcliffe to show how grateful they were. 'I said, they've been so amazing with you. We need to show how much we value them.'

Someone suggested a marathon. A place came up in the 2007 London race. There was little time to prepare, but a friend who ran – actually the daughter of one of those lifelong friends mentioned earlier – reassured her that, if nothing else, she could walk it. In fact, she ran, 'chatting all the way' and 'loving every minute' – and finished in just under four hours. It was two days after her sixtieth birthday.

Her young friend, incredulous, urged her to visit her running club. She did, and was won over by its friendly atmosphere. Rugby & Northampton AC embraces a wide range of age groups, including a handful of runners of around Angela's age. 'I started to think: "This is all right to do this"' – whereas previously she had feared that people would think it 'really odd to see an old person running'. Thursday evening club nights became a cherished part of her week.

Soon she was racing too – her club-mates insisted she try it. She felt awkward at first, lining up at the start with lots of women forty years younger than her. In fact, initially she preferred to hang around inconspicuously at the back. But after a couple of races 'I became quite competitive', and soon she was jostling for the best starting position along with everyone else.

She was regularly the winner in her age group, usually at distances from 5 miles to half-marathon, and before 2007 was out she had set four records, including a W60 world record for the half-marathon. But that was just her warm-up. The following year she won her first British Masters title, in the W60 cross-country, and was introduced to a highly respected local coach, Ian Wilson, who became her mentor and good friend. She was, he told me once, a difficult athlete to coach, because 'she races far too much.' ('But I enjoy it,' protested Copson. 'It's a sociable thing . . .') On the other hand, she had that raw talent that every coach dreams of finding. In one of her first British championship finals, she accidentally stopped a lap early in the 5,000m. Ian had to shout at her to run another lap – 'but she still set a world record.'

Ian, who sadly died of cancer in December 2020, helped Copson to become not just a winner but an unstoppable force in international Masters athletics. In 2012, she went to her first European Masters championships, in Zittau, Germany. A W65 by then, she won four golds and was later named European Masters Woman Athlete of the Year.

Her subsequent dominance of her age groups has been overwhelming. She is the oldest woman ever to break three-and-a-half hours for a marathon (3:24:54, a few days before her sixty-ninth birthday). In 2018, at the World Masters in Málaga, she won seven golds (and a bronze), while in May 2019, aged seventy-two, she won the Westminster Masters Mile in 6:27, knocking over a minute off the British W70 record for a road mile and eleven-and-a-half seconds off the world track record. Her age grading score for that race was an almost unprecedented 107.2 per cent.

She had by then already been awarded a British Empire Medal for 'services to running', and by 2021 her career tally of records and medals included thirty-seven world records, fifty European records, seventy-two British records and 146 championship medals, at distances from 400m to marathon, including twenty world golds. But even she is losing count. 'I just put them in a shoebox and forget about them.' And if you're tempted to think, ah, but medals and records in the oldest age groups are just a matter of turning up, think again. These are serious times. Her W65 bests included 5:30.7 for 1500m; 20:13.23 for 5,000m; 41:40.27 for 10,000m; and 3 hours 17 minutes for the marathon. Her W70 equivalents are 5:46.90, 20:56.13, 44:25.14 and 3:36:30. How many of those times would *you* be confident of beating?

She could, in many of her races, run quite a lot slower and still win. She has plenty of gifted and committed rivals, but – like LeClerc and Nakano – Copson has that special extraordinary something that, in younger age-groups, separates the podium-bound Olympic super-elite by a huge margin from the best recreational enthusiasts. I have seen her open up a forty-metre lead before the first bend of a middle-distance race, and win by well over a lap. That doesn't make her achievements worth less. It emphasises how special she is.

When Copson went to EMAC-Venice in September

2019 they held a dinner in her honour. 'It was lovely,' she says casually, but she didn't stay for long. She has, she says, grown used to being treated as a sporting phenomenon, but sometimes she feels 'hammered' by all the media requests, and she would never think of herself as a celebrity. Instead she remains, at heart, that same almost accidental runner, who stumbled into the sport – just as millions of others in similar positions have done – on the back of a charitable impulse. When she started, she used to go out for her serious training runs after dark, 'so that no one would see me'.

She's more confident now – how could she not be? – but her sense of running's proper place in the world hasn't changed. She does it because she loves to feel fit and strong, and because – lockdowns permitting – she loves the sport's social side. And if she ever reaches a stage where she can no longer compete, 'I'll always jog along,' she says.

Yet for all the unexpected joy and adventure that running has brought to her life over the past fifteen years or so, she insists that 'it doesn't come first. Family does.' No matter how bold her record-breaking goals, she'll happily skip a race or a run to spend time with her grandchildren, and if she puts time and thought into preparing healthy meals, that's for Harry's benefit as much as hers. She doesn't see her sporting ambitions as a reason to deprive herself of little pleasures such as wine or cake, and even the most prestigious championships take second place to loved ones at home. In 2019 she limited her involvement in EMAC-Venice because of family commitments, and concern for her husband's well-being meant that, even if it hadn't been cancelled, she would probably have missed the 2020 World Masters in Toronto. 'He's really not into long flights any more, and I feel a bit selfish just going off and not including him.'

I don't think it's fanciful to speculate that this sense of balance and proportion has influenced Copson's running. Her movements on the track are balanced and flowing, with little sign of stiffness or tension, and although she's tiny – just 5ft 1in – she always seems too grounded to be frail. And it is in this, now I think of it, that she most resembles LeClerc and Nakano. All three seem liberated when they run: grateful to be there, even when pushing against the limits of endurance. They are naturals – which makes it all the more sobering to think how close they came to never discovering running at all.

But in that, at least, they are not unusual. The world is full of elderly women who never got a chance to explore their athletic potential when they were young. Most don't do so when they are old, either: hence those vast winning margins – although that is, I hope, starting to change.

Meanwhile, it is hard for the ageing male runner not to feel humbled, as well as inspired, by what Copson, LeClerc and Nakano have accomplished. Men of my generation were taught to associate toughness with maleness. All our lives, we have been encouraged to 'man up': in sport, in the workplace, in everyday life. Some of us have even been reprimanded for acting 'like an old woman'. So it is salutary to be reminded, by the evidence of our own eyes, how wildly inappropriate such language is.

In fact, if there is a 'weaker sex' when it comes to resilience and general endurance, it is men. It's the male mid-life crisis, not the female one, that traditionally provokes melodramatic over-reaction. Women get the menopause; we get a Harley-Davidson and run off with a foreign woman half our age. But the self-congratulatory myth of male toughness is, I think, part of the problem, encouraging us to pretend, to ourselves and to our rivals, that we are weakness-free. This often helps us, in the short term. In the long term, it is unsustainable. The hidden damage, physical and emotional, accumulates, unacknowledged and unresolved, until one day, just as we are making the mid-life shift from 'young' to 'old', life confronts us with the awful truth: not only are we not the men we used to be, but we were never the men we pretended to be. We are imperfect beings, vulnerable creatures who from now on will increasingly be defined by our physical weaknesses; beings whose essence is to be damaged, worn-out and torn. That's hard to take, when you've spent most of your life acting the part of a superhero – and valuing yourself accordingly. Hence all those existential crises. We cannot bear to think of ourselves as damaged goods.

But women tend to lead less sheltered lives, where discouragement is concerned. All those things that come as a nasty, identity-threatening shock to the older man – being talked over and ignored, undervalued and underpaid: women have often been soaking up such slights for years, usually while shouldering more than their fair share of family responsibilities. Women are also likely to be fatalistically familiar with the agonies of childbirth, and with the trials of living in a body that puts the imperatives of reproduction ahead of their own needs. In short, they tend to face up sooner than men to the fact that life is less than ideal, and develop the habit of responding in the only appropriate way: by getting over it, getting on with it and making the best of it. Even the final injustice – that women are more likely than men to be left bereaved by the loss of a long-term partner – fits into this pattern. There is nothing to be done about it, except, somehow, to bear it. But elderly widows have at least had some practice. As women, they are used to life's unfairness; and this has often given them a particular strength: the habit of not breaking, and enduring whatever has to be endured.

For other runners in their age group, Copson, LeClerc and Nakano are superheroes, as awesome and enviable as Olympians. Yet the heroes themselves see it differently. They are simply getting on with their lives, without fuss, just as they have always done, while relishing experiences that they never got the chance to enjoy when they were young, and making the best of them. That's why the same concepts keep coming up in our conversations: 'gratitude'; 'adventure'; 'discovery'. And that, I think, is what runners of any gender can most helpfully learn from them.

But the achievements of the record-breaking latecomers also suggest a more subtle lesson. Taking up competitive running in old age isn't just an adventure. It can also be experienced as a kind of liberation, because it allows us to reclaim the right to be the people we choose to be. Few of us get beyond retirement age without being placed in limiting conceptual boxes. Society labels us as 'old', 'frail', 'past it' or 'vulnerable', and our worlds shrink to match. Yet those of us who are lucky enough to remain relatively active and mobile can, if we wish, choose our own label: as active athletes, with exciting goals.

For some women, there can be the surprising relief that, thanks to their age, the world may at last have stopped judging them against stereotypes of supposed wifely or motherly duty. For the first time since child-hood they find that they can revel unselfconsciously in their bodies' physical potential, and often feel less tyrannised by the sexually objectifying male gaze. As Kathrine Switzer put it in her 1998 book, *Running and Walking for Women Over Forty*, 'Shedding the pressures and expectations of youth allows you to be yourself . . . This sense of freedom can make you soar.' This is one of the things that makes Alex Rotas's photographs so joyful: her subjects' grey hairs, lined faces, papery skin and time-worn teeth give them the free-dom to be themselves; and that creates a beauty far richer than mere youthful flawlessness.

It would be facile to deny the reality of late life's pains and sorrows. But the freedom it brings is real too. Being old means no longer having to pretend – to be tougher than we are, for example, or more desirable. Instead, we can be ourselves – which for many of us is a slightly unfa-miliar experience. And if we are runners and are lucky enough not to have been immobilised by physiological decay, we can also run as ourselves, weaknesses and all, chasing our dreams, realistic or improbable, without embarrassment. All it takes is to accept that the past is gone; that we are damaged creatures; that our remaining time is finite; and that what's left of life is for the living.

21

Reach for the stars

I decided that I needed a dream. All those stories of late-life hope and resilience had left me restless, with envy and admiration. Now it was time to stop being a mere fan and begin a running adventure of my own.

I resolved to set my sights high. After all, I told myself, Yoko Nakono was a total beginner when she was my age. So was Angela Copson. They had no more running achievements to their name than I have – and now look at them. Why, then, should my undistinguished athletic record limit my ambitions?

I also believed, at that point, that significant improvement was within my reach, thanks to my most comprehensive counter-attack against ageing so far. For several weeks now, I had been focusing on running basics: balance, economy, range and fluency of motion; full and appropriate engagement of every muscle and tendon. Gone were the days of tacking a few anti-ageing extras on to my existing training routines. Now I did it the other way round. Some days felt like extended sessions of rehabilitative physiotherapy. I did mobilisation exercises, balance exercises, stability exercises, resistance exercises. I did sit-ups, press-ups, planks; and squats, on two legs and on one. I worked my adductors and abductors, too, and my lower abdominals, and I spent hours trying to loosen my seized-up ankles and hips. What running I did was slow, over short distances – there was no time for more – and most of the effort went into trying not to cut biomechanical corners. My mileage plummeted; so, I imagine, did my cardiovascular fitness. Yet I sensed that I was making progress. I was stronger, if not faster; and when I did run, I often did so without pain.

I had been trying to be more intelligent about fuelling my body, too – although whether that meant cutting back radically on carbohydrate or doing the opposite depended on which specialist I consulted. I had been trying, belatedly, to guard against over-eating (an increasing hazard as the ageing runner's metabolism slows down), while also being wary of under-eating (an increasing hazard as our deteriorating sense of taste reduces our appetite and our ability to absorb nutrients declines). I had increased my intake of protein (vital for fighting sarcopenia) and now made sure that I always consumed some of it – typically as nuts – within fifteen minutes or so of finishing training. (Leave it much longer and you don't get the full benefit.) I had also been making a conscious effort to keep up my water intake – because ageing reduces our sensitivity to thirst. I had even overturned my decades-old preference for running on an empty stomach, persuaded by an expert consensus that older runners who want to maintain and rebuild their running muscles need to train with fuel inside them (for glucose availability), especially when training intensely.

Those are just the edited highlights of a science-based re-set of my daily habits that would, I hoped, dramatically increase my chances of ageing slowly over the coming decades. I could have done with such an overhaul long ago; and I sensed that I would need to keep this up conscientiously for several years before my body felt the full benefits. I couldn't help noticing, however, that it wasn't a whole lot of fun.

All that sensible behaviour required conscious thought and, often, quite a lot of time; and it went on day after day after day. It wasn't difficult, and the under-lying science seemed sound, but where was the joy or the buzz? It reminded me of all those doomed New Year's resolutions I used to make as a young man: stop drinking; stop smoking; stop gambling; get a career. Yes, of course. But how do you get fired up about being sensible?

Never mind, I had been telling myself this time round. You don't need to be fired up. All that matters is that you stick at it, avoid injury, and end each week a slightly stronger runner than you were when it began. Focus on that, and in due course you'll get your reward.

Yet without a dream, that reasoning seemed laughable. What was this imagined reward? To shuffle along obscurely at a slightly less pathetic pace than would otherwise have been the case? It barely felt worth the extra trouble.

So I started to think about a big goal to set myself: a pie-in-the-sky target that would fire me up with enthusiasm. Otherwise, an injury might close this rare window of runner's luck before I had made the most of it, and all I would be left with was dutiful damage limitation.

The goal needed to be just about achievable, or I wouldn't believe in it; but it didn't need to be sensible. After all, I reminded myself, Gene Dykes took 34 minutes off his marathon time between the ages of sixty-five and seventy, while Alan Carter took 14 seconds off his 400m time in the year leading up to his first international race as a seventy-year-old. Who knows what I might achieve, if everything went right? Even if a really spectacular improvement was beyond me, I might none the less become a significantly better runner. And in the meantime I could at least re-familiarise myself with the thrill – which younger runners take for granted – of training in pursuit of my utmost physical limits.

What should I dream of, though? A running goal can be your daily companion for months, sometimes years, so there needs to be a romantic spark. I mused through the options. A marathon? I'd done marathons, and had never felt much affection for the distance. A sub-three-hour marathon? That did excite me, but did it tick the 'achievable' box? (No.)

What about an ultra, or some kind of big, remote adventure race? Many late-life runners find such events motivating; some seem rejuvenated by them. Yet I couldn't find one that I felt like sharing a big chunk of my life with. I spent much of my thirties and forties pushing myself to the limits of my endurance in wild, mountainous places (as described in my 2004 book, *Feet in the Clouds*), and I felt I had already made the most of what limited talent I had for that kind of running. I will never lose my love of running on fells and trails, at whatever speed I can comfortably manage. But an extreme, soul-testing challenge that would define my life for months? I'd done that.

It also struck me that, if I wanted a real adventure, I should look outside my habitual comfort zones. This implied a challenge involving speed, not stamina – which again seemed to rule out the traditional mid-life ultra.

And that's when my dream began to take shape. Anyone

can keep going for mile after mountainous mile, I told myself. Toughness, when you're older, is running hard and fast against the clock. That's who the real superheroes of late-life running are: the champions of track-and-field. (Even Ed Whitlock set more world records on the track than on the road.) In which case, if I wanted to find my own inner hero – which is basically what recreational running goals are about – I needed to find a way of somehow running in their footsteps, or perhaps even experiencing the same challenges as them.

After that, the dream took on its own momentum. My imagination wrapped the core of good sense in layer after layer of increasingly extravagant fantasy, and before long I had a wild, extravagant plan: to try my luck at an international track-and-field championship.

I kept all this to myself. Obviously. It was ludicrous. But every now and then one of my world-beating interviewees would ask me about my own running aspirations; and every now and then I would let slip little hints, to the effect that, well, maybe when I was considerably fitter I wouldn't mind testing myself against a slightly higher standard – perhaps even at, er, international level.

And then one day, when I was talking to Steve Peters, he picked up on the hint and said: 'Are you going to be running in Finland, then?'

Finland, in this context, meant the 2022 World Masters Athletics Championships in Tampere, Finland, and – just in case I haven't already made this obvious – it was absurd that I should even be thinking of competing at such an event. It would be like wangling my way into the starting line-up of a Premier League football team: an adventure, undeniably, but mainly a cringe-making embarrassment.

'Yes,' I said. 'I think so.'

To my surprise, he didn't laugh. 'That would be great,' said Peters. 'You should do it. I think it's great that more people come into it. Have a go!'

I explained that I really would be way, way off the pace – almost anti-socially so.

'I don't think it's wise to compare,' he said. 'What's interesting is: "Did I do my best?" Do it for yourself. If you run your best and that's your best, then great.' Then he told me about some of the runners he comes up against: people whose personal best is equivalent to his warm-up pace, or 'guys I train with, and all they want is to make the second round, or, you know, maybe just beat one other person. I really admire that. I really appreciate them being on the track with me.'

Jo Pavey didn't laugh either. 'That would be great,' she echoed. 'Trying to do all these different things that we do to combat ageing, it can just end up with you being more injured. But if you have a goal, you can prioritise. So you need to ask yourself: right, what are the specific things I need to do to achieve what I want to achieve in my event?'

It had emerged by then that the most suitable event for someone like me to enter in Tampere would be the 10km road race: not quite the short sharp track event I had originally had in mind, but at least one in which I could blend in at the back of the field, among the W80s and M90s, without causing inconvenience or offence.

So Jo's advice focused on her own experience of knocking herself into championship shape for the 10,000m, notably in 2014, when she had to get her forty-year-old body back into medal-winning shape for the European Championships, within months of giving birth to her second child. Her approach, she explained, was to turn her age into a positive. 'When I was younger, I used to think, right, an athlete needs to do this, and this, and this. And I ended up being injured for two and a half years. But this time I knew what I needed. So rather than going out and doing miles and miles and miles, I kept doing interval sessions. I did as many track sessions as I could get away with as long as there was two days' easy running in between. And I just kept repeating that. I did enough strength and conditioning for core stability, but I didn't do anything that could potentially make my legs bad for a track session. I kept thinking, time's up against me, and I knew from experience that I needed to hit certain times for k-reps, 400m, 800m, to have any chance. But that's where age helps. You're better at listening to your body and putting together a training mix.'

In my case, she reckoned, if I wanted to run 10km at a higher level, I needed a similar approach. 'You don't need to run for miles and miles. But you do need to train for speed. Otherwise you'll blow up after one kilometre. So prioritise the main things, but listen to your body and give yourself the chance of recovery.'

The individual speed sessions needed to be adaptable too, so that I could steer the right course between too little and too much: 'You need to stretch yourself. But it shouldn't be so full out that you feel destroyed afterwards. It's more important to do it regularly, focusing on running form and the extra leg-power you're generating. Afterwards you might feel a bit sore, but then later you start feeling that you're getting more spring off your legs.'

So that, over the coming weeks, was what I did. I found

a field, a fifteen-minute jog from my home, that was generally empty first thing in the morning. It's a big, gently steepening slope of rough pasture, occasionally grazed by sheep, with a straightish semblance of a grassy path trodden straight up through the middle. I've never measured it exactly, but it's about 400m from bottom to top, give or take various wiggles and boggy patches, and if you run it briskly even once you really notice how the gradient grows crueller towards the end. It was no good for a proper athlete – sorry, a serious athlete – but for my purposes it was fine. The surface was forgiving (for now) and, over time, I used it to reacquaint myself with the sensation of running hard and fast. Later, I found that I could really torture myself with repetitions, keeping up a rhythm even when my lungs were screaming for rest, then using the gentle downhill jog for recovery. There was no science to it, but anything that hurt that much must have been doing me some good. And for four or five successive weeks in the spring of 2022 I kept going back to that field, whenever I felt that my body could take it.

That wasn't particularly often. I had other pressures in my life, and not many recent miles in my legs, and there were many mornings when I felt that I just needed to be gentle with myself. But at least I didn't go backwards. My injury-free streak was several months old, and I could feel myself getting stronger. My body seemed to want to run hard again. My confidence improved. And when I varied my regime with a bit of road-running (since I needed to get used to running on tarmac again) and suffered from sore knees afterwards, I was amazed to find that, twenty-four hours later, my knees were almost miraculously pain-free. Maybe, finally, things were getting better; and if I kept this up, who knows? Maybe I could get back some of the things age had stolen from me: my power, my speed, my elasticity, my resilience; all the things that had once made me a decent runner.

Then I did what Steve Peters had specifically advised me not to do.

I hadn't initially intended to compare myself with anybody. I just wanted to check a couple of Angela Copson's records. But before I knew it I was browsing through the WMA world record lists in their entirety – male and female, right through the age groups. If I wanted to compete internationally, I told myself, I needed to know what the standards were at the top. 'Don't compare,' Peters had warned. But of course I did compare, and within fifteen minutes I was almost weeping with demoralisation. For example: the all-time best by an M60 at 10,000m, recorded by Japan's Yoshitsugu Iwanaga in November 2020, is 33:39.52. This seemed barely comprehensible. There are runners in the world – Uganda's Olympic champion, Joshua Cheptegei, for example – who could run an entire 5,000m race in less time than the gap between Yoshitugu's record and my time on the Wimbledon Park track. We might as well be doing different sports.

Crushed, I kept browsing, hoping to find gentler comparisons. All I found were bigger, more humiliating gulfs. By the time I gave up, it was too late. I had no self-belief left: just a gut-wrenching embarrassment at my deluded sense that I could ever be any good as a late-life runner. Perhaps you'll feel something similar, if you take a look at this small but loosely representative selection of a few world bests (as of 2022) in some of the older age groups.

M60: 100m: 11.70; 200m: 24.00; 400m: 53.88; 800m: 2:08.56; 1500m: 4:24.00; 5000m: 15:56.41; 10,000m: 33:39.52; marathon: 2:30:02.

W60: 100m: 13.20; 200m: 27.78; 400m: 1:04.31; 800m: 2:31.51; 1500m: 5:06.65; 5000m: 17:59.16; 10,000m: 37:57.95; marathon: 2:52:13.

M70: 100m: 12.77; 200m: 25.75; 400m: 57.26; 800m: 2:20.52; 1500m: 4:52.95; 5000m: 18:15.53; 10,000m: 38:04.13; marathon: 2:54:19.

W70: 100m: 14.73; 200m: 31.30; 400m: 1:12.76; 800m: 2:50.66; 1500m: 5:46.9; 5000m: 20:56.13; 10,000m: 44:25.14; marathon: 3:28:46.

M80: 100m: 14.35; 200m: 29.54; 400m: 1:10.01; 800m: 2:41.59; 1500m: 5:30.89; 5000m: 20:20.01; 10,000m: 42:39.95; marathon: 3:15:54.

W80: 100m: 16.26; 200m: 35.34; 400m: 1:29.84; 800m: 3:30.41; 1500m: 6:52.77; 5000m: 25:40.14; 10,000m: 51:46.65; marathon: 4:11:45.

M90: 100m: 16.86; 200m: 36.02; 400m: 1:29.15; 800m: 3:34.93; 1500m: 7:32.95 5000m: 29:59.94; 10,000m: 1:02:48.93 marathon: 5:40:03.

W90: 100m: 23.15; 200m: 55.62; 400m: 2:16.19; 800m: 5:01.35; 1500m: 12:34.67; 5000m: 54:46.35; marathon: 7:03:59. (There is no official W90 record for running 10,000m, but the 10km race-walk world record of 1:25:28 will probably do for our purposes.)

These are very incomplete lists, in terms of events as well as age categories, and no doubt several of the records will have been broken by the time you read this. Yet the overall impression they give is fair. This is what the heights of late-life athletic achievement look like.

For me, and I suspect most runners, those heights are dizzyingly out of reach. There isn't enough sports science in the solar system to get me remotely near Iwanaga's standard, or Tommy Hughes's, or (still less) that of Ron Taylor, the British sprinter whose M60 100m and 200m records have stood since 1994. The levels of achievement are breathtaking, right across the age groups, for women as well as for men. It's tempting to give up.

So that's what I did. I had no more business racing in a world championships as a sixty-two-year-old than I would have had competing in the Olympics as a twenty-two-year-old. My dream was just middle-aged fantasy; whereas what I needed was to grow up and give up.

Then, within a day, I changed my mind. I had to keep going, or all my previous efforts would have been wasted. In any case, what's so good about growing up? It's too little dreaming that turns our lives grey, not too much, and it's all those decades of acting grown-up that make it happen. At least my fantasy gave me a goal.

So I picked up the training routines I had set myself, even as part of my mind protested that I was merely throwing good money after bad. Maybe there's a point to all this, I told myself, even if it takes me nowhere. At least it must be making me healthier, and more resistant to age-related decay. But what I really wanted was a bit more hope in my heart, and a bit more faith in my dream.

22

Running brave

The weeks went by. I stuck to my smart-ish, age-focused training routines, dutifully rather than passionately. And I began to sense that, despite my doubts, I was becoming more resilient; or, at least, marginally less pathetic. Physical toughness remained elusive, and race-ready fitness came and went. Yet my setbacks no longer filled me with despair. I took them in my stride. And sometimes it even seemed that they were making me stronger.

This was an unexpected paradox, yet it felt significant. I had a good idea by now of what I needed to do. I also knew that, if I added it all up (easy runs, tempo runs, speed sessions, proper warm-ups, cross-training, strength work, exercises for balance, stability and mobility, plyometric hopping and jumping, careful meal planning, rehabilitative physio and, not least, lots of rest, recovery and sleep) it came to a hell of a lot. And I knew that, most weeks, much of it wasn't going to happen. I had other things to focus on, and there was a limit to how much I could sanely neglect work, family, community and home, just for the sake of a hobby I'm only moderately good at (or not even that, in the light of those records).

This didn't bode well for my aspirations in Finland. Yet

facing up to it proved unexpectedly empowering. It forced me, for a start, to focus on essentials. I knew I couldn't stick consistently to any recognised system or formula. But I had, I think, hit on something valuable when I told myself to remember the three 'mores': more recovery; more intensity; more patience. Not all at once, obviously, but as loose, recurring rules, which, over time, moulded my training. I thought, too, about Steve Peters, 'slowly building' if he did three of his sessions a week but 'weakening' if he did only two. And I tried to keep in mind Nick Lauder's advice: 'Rule number one of Masters Athletics is: don't get injured. And rule number two is: don't forget rule number one.' All this hardly amounted to a training programme, but taken together it seemed to give me a sensible framework for improvement.

But there was also something more important. I realised that falling short was now so hard-wired into my running life that it had become a given. There was no point denying it, or pretending I could eliminate all my failings. I simply wasn't the runner I would ideally wish to be – and I never would be. But this, of course, is true for every Masters runner. The days of unlimited possibility are gone. And what I was finally grasping was that late-life athletes who thrive are those who have made their peace with reality. They know that perfection isn't an option, only damage limitation.

The more this sank in – and it would have been hard to spend so much time interacting with Masters athletes without absorbing much of it – the more I found myself making my peace with other truths. Life is a mess; most things are beyond our control; things tend to deteriorate. All we can do is empower ourselves to be strong by facing up to our weakness; and try, in the timeless formula expressed by John Keston (the British-American actor, author, singer and record-breaking Masters runner who died, aged ninety-seven, in 2022), to 'keep moving, and be kind to people.'

It's strange that it took me so long to understand all this, because these are central facts of late-life running. Every Masters athlete is a damaged athlete. Even the champions – those superb specimens of late-life manhood and womanhood I had previously contemplated only with envy – have fought their own losing battles against age, bitterly conceding ground over many years to physiological decay and life's random cruelties. Their biggest triumph is in remaining unbroken.

'Just getting to the starting line is a miracle of some sort,' argues Ken Stone, the US journalist and blogger, talking about his fascination with older Masters. 'They've been through divorces, deaths, illnesses, careers ending; they've been buffeted by the economy. That's what makes them so interesting.' I had reached a similar conclusion, and was belatedly drawing my own lessons from it. What I really ought to be thinking about my own little struggles as a runner wasn't how hard it all was but how lucky I was – to be still running and still struggling. And what I ought to envy about the supreme exponents of the sport wasn't their athletic prowess but their courage and grit.

Some of the all-time greats of late-life running have come through trials and tragedies that make all my runner's woes and self-pity seem grotesquely self-indulgent. They have endured the seemingly unendurable. And it is for that, rather than the medals they won or the records they set, that they are venerated as giants of their sport.

John Gilmour, who died in 2018 at the age of ninety-nine, was a notable example. When he disembarked in Fremantle, Western Australia, at the end of the Second World War, he was a twenty-six-year-old lance-corporal, and he had to be helped off the ship. He had put on a pound or two on the slow voyage from Japan, but he still weighed only 6st 6lb. His eyesight had been permanently damaged by malnutrition. On the bright side, he said, he couldn't see the look on his mother's face when she saw him.

Before the war, Gilmour, a factory worker, had been one of Western Australia's strongest distance runners, with dreams of competing at a higher level. But three years as a prisoner-of-war and slave labourer in Singapore and Japan – including fifteen months in the notorious Changi prison – had wrecked him physically. Only his spirit was undamaged.

He had kept himself going in captivity with the thought that, one day, he would run again, properly. After a spell in hospital, he did. His doctor advised against it, but Gilmour had learnt to believe in himself. He had had to. Within a year, despite being partially blind, he won the West Australian Ten Mile Road Racing Championship. It was too late for any hopes of becoming an Olympian, but he continued, gradually, to regain his strength, and he won several more regional and national titles before hanging up his running shoes in 1956. He was thirty-seven, with a family and a full-time job as a hospital gardener. There wasn't a lot of time for athletics, and what time there was went into setting up a local club and coaching young athletes there.

Then, in 1962, the Commonwealth Games were held in Perth, his local city. The excitement of the spectacle re-awakened his competitive hunger. He decided to try for a place in the state marathon team for the Australian championships. He reached the necessary standard but wasn't selected – apparently because, at forty-three, he was too old. So when a friend introduced him to Masters athletics a few years later, he flung himself into it delightedly. He had unfinished sporting business.

His career in Masters lasted nearly half a century. He was part of a small party of visiting Australians who competed in David Pain's US Masters championships in San Diego in July 1971 – and set his first two world records there. By the time he ran his last race, at the world championships in Perth in 2016, he had set more than a hundred world records in different Masters age groups, and was admired internationally as a figurehead of the movement. He estimated that he had competed in more than 1,000 races, including more than twenty marathons. His achievements included a 2:38:19 marathon as a fifty-nine-year-old (which theoretically qualified him for selection for the Olympics) and a 38:49.25 10,000m as a seventy-year-old. But he was also revered for the dignity with which he eventually returned to compete as a Master in both Japan and Singapore. 'The Japanese veterans seemed more intent on encouraging me than concentrating on their own performance,' he enthused.

All this, remember, while partially blind, which somehow didn't prevent him from training up to 100 miles a week until well into his fifties. There were falls, in competition as well as training. 'Not being able to see is definitely a handicap in running,' he conceded. But 'I'd tell myself: "Get up, Gilmour. In no way is running a race going to defeat you after what you've been through."'

As the years went by, he fell more often. There was a serious road accident in the early 1980s, and a nasty dog attack in 2001. Injuries and illness weakened him, and he never entirely shook off the after-effects of those wartime years of torture and starvation. But he was never heard to complain. He just picked himself up and started again.

In 2005 he retired from athletics to look after his sick wife, Alma. He said he wanted her to know that, despite all his previous sporting travels, 'I thought more of her than my running.' But Alma died in 2012, and when Perth was chosen to host the World Masters Athletics Championships of 2016, Gilmour realised he still had a bit more running to do.

He was ninety-seven when the Games came round, and almost totally blind. He trained by running round his house and garden: either 80-metre circuits of the whole property, or 25-metre laps of a soft earth track he had made in his back yard. He tried to do two or three kilometres a day. 'I have yet to burn out,' he said once. 'Burning out is in your mind, through listening to others talking instead of your own body. You burn out when you're looking for an excuse.'

He ran his last two races with a urostomy bag attached to his left leg. The first event, at 800m, took him 9:19.93. His last race of all, at 1500m, took 19:35.95. He won gold for both, being the only M95 competitor in either race. In each case, there was an M90 to race against: Romania's Dumitru Radu in the 800m and China's Zhiyong Wang in the 1500m. And in each case he finished to a spine-tingling standing ovation.

'This is not athletics,' said Alan Bell, the race director, afterwards. 'This is more an example of the human spirit.'

Actually I think he was wrong. Gilmour's unbreakable spirit was at some level inseparable from his running. His refusal to surrender to his physical limitations as an athlete was a source of strength in his broader rejection of despair. Running topped up his courage.

A similar interplay between the challenges of running and the challenges of surviving as an unbroken human being can be seen in the story of Ida Keeling. You could, if you chose, tell her story in exclusively sporting terms – and it wouldn't take long. Towards the end of her life, the US sprinter set world records in the W90, W95 and W100 age groups. These were also the first official race times recorded by a woman in those categories. In August 2021, she died, aged 106. The end.

To understand her story, however, you need to know about the decades of suffering and loss that preceded her achievements on the track.

Ida Keeling was born in May 1915 to immigrant parents (from the Virgin Islands), the second of eight children, and raised in the notorious Manhattan slum district known as Hell's Kitchen. They were evicted from their home on the eve of the Great Depression, and all ten of them ended up living at the back of their one remaining asset, a small grocery store. Later, they lost that too. Ida's mother died around the same time, and Ida, still in her teens, found herself in partial charge of her younger siblings. She did what she could to better herself, studying for a while at the Textile High School in the nearby Chelsea district, but couldn't afford to complete her course.

For the next fifty years she worked uncomplainingly in a long series of menial jobs, often in garment factories.

But the setbacks kept coming. Her first fiancée turned out to be married already. She had two sons before she found out. At one point, she and the boys spent nearly a year living in a homeless shelter.

Her second marriage was blighted by her husband's alcohol abuse. Divorce was imminent when he died suddenly, aged forty-two. Ida was thirty-eight and now had two daughters as well as two sons. To make ends meet, she moved three of her children into a one-bedroom apartment in central Harlem, in a housing project soon to be notorious for gangs and violence and, from the 1960s, drugs. In the Navy her eldest son, Donald, developed his own drug habit, and then drifted, to Ida's distress, into the orbit of their good-for-nothing father. Charles, the youngest, soon followed a similar trajectory. But Laura and Shelley, Ida's daughters, stayed with her, and she, to support them, juggled her work between multiple employers: the Department of Motor Vehicles, Harlem Hospital, various restaurants and factories. All through the 1960s and 1970s, she rarely had fewer than two jobs on the go. Well-paid work for poor, black women simply wasn't a thing in New York back then.

The more Ida saw of the world, the more social injustice bothered her. In August 1963, she was among the 250,000 marchers who heard Martin Luther King's most famous speech at the Lincoln Memorial, Washington. Most of the time she was too busy to do more than dream of change, but her daughters did well for themselves – Shelley, the youngest, became a lawyer and an athletics coach – and when Ida retired in 1977, aged sixty-two, she had reason to believe that the struggles and stresses of her hard life were coming to an end.

Instead, in 1978, Donald was murdered – hanged, in the stairwell of a tenement building, apparently as retribution for a drug deal gone wrong. In late 1980, Charles was murdered too: beaten to death with a baseball bat. Like his brother, he had clearly strayed too deeply into the world of the drug gangs.

'It just broke me,' Ida admitted when we spoke towards the end of her life. 'I was in such a deep hole . . .'

'A light had gone off inside her,' says Shelley today. Ida put on weight; her blood pressure soared; for two years, she barely went out: just sat at home watching soap operas. 'It felt like I was moving around in a bowl of thick oatmeal,' Ida wrote later. 'It was all I could do to reach out and change the channel on my TV set.'

But life wasn't finished with her. One day, in September 1982, Shelley dropped in. She could no longer bear to watch her mother fall apart. So she told Ida she needed a favour: 'I need you to go to a cross-country race with me.' Shelley had been a keen runner for several years, so Ida assumed she was required as a spectator. Then Shelley explained: 'No, I want you to run.'

The race she had in mind was a 5km 'mini run' in Brooklyn a few days later. The idea seemed so preposterous Ida couldn't find the energy to protest. By the day of the race, however, she had come up with the excuse that she didn't have any running shoes. Shelley forestalled that by producing a pair from her bag. Ida objected that they felt too tight. Shelley produced an alternative pair.

And so it was that this heartbroken sixty-seven-year-old, sunk in misery but fresh out of excuses, found herself on a starting-line with 200 other runners and set off for the first race of her life. She was easily the oldest and was soon so far behind that she felt 'like a little tugboat'.

She was thinking of giving up when the idea came into her head that 'maybe this is good for me'. So she kept going, slowly, noticing the contrast between her running and her day-to-day depression and telling herself: 'I got to get out of this rut, I got to get out of this rut.' And then, she told Shelley later, she began to feel as though she was running up and out of a hole – 'like someone had watered a plant that had not been watered in a long time'. By the finish: 'I felt so different. I felt free. My mind wasn't on my troubles.'

After a while, she tried another run, and then another and another. She joined a running club. She noticed how, each time she ran, the movements caused her to feel relaxed and uplifted – 'like I'm out with the wind', she once said. In short: she discovered that she was a runner. Without that change of identity, she wrote later, she would soon have been dead, or at best would 'have a quality of life so low, it wouldn't matter if I was alive'. Instead, she picked herself up and, as time went by, her surviving family sensed her inner light returning.

She was far from being a champion in those early years: she was just another road runner, trying to run off her troubles like the rest of us. But her life was still a work in progress. In 1995, she turned eighty, and was persuaded to try her luck on the track at the World Masters Championships in Buffalo, New York. She ran 800m and, although she didn't win, she loved the experience. Thereafter, she became a track athlete, and she quickly realised that what she really liked was sprinting. 'I wanted to go as fast as I could.'

Gradually, simply by sticking at it, Ida became

remarkable. In 2008, Shelley took her mother to France for the World Masters Games in Clermont-Ferrand. Shelley was competing herself, as a W55 at 400m, and Ida, then ninety-two, was persuaded to race at 60m. She won unopposed, in 31.82 seconds, and her time became the first ever W90 world record at the distance.

Meanwhile, Ida had moved out of Harlem, first to Queens and then to the Bronx, where she lived, mostly alone, for nearly twenty years. Far from being lonely, however, she became a minor celebrity, with public interest in her achievements increasing with each new birthday. In 2011, at New York's Armory Track and Field Center in Manhattan, she set another world record for 60m, this time as a ninety-five-year-old. Her time was 29.86: faster than her previous record. But she was in any case the first W95 to record an official time for the distance. A year or so later, aged ninety-seven, she set another W95 world record – 51.85 seconds for 100m – at the USATF Eastern Regional Conference Championships. Two years after that, at the 2014 Gay Games in Akron, Ohio, she ran the same distance slightly slower, in 59.80. It was, however, both the fastest and the only time yet recorded for a ninety-nine-year-old woman.

Each of these achievements prompted a fresh burst of media interest, and by the time Ida turned a hundred she was a national figure. Every network television chat show seemed to want her as a guest, and when ABC filmed a series of short statements from some of America's most admired female figures to celebrate Hillary Clinton's expected victory in the 2016 presidential election, Ida – a lifelong Democrat – was one of those chosen. (Hillary, however, wasn't . . .)

Earlier that year, just short of her 101st birthday, Ida had raced in front of 44,469 spectators at the Penn Relays meet in Philadelphia. She wasn't the only runner in the 100m race, which mixed genders and age groups, and she finished a distant last, in 1 minute 17.33 seconds. But the applause, specifically for her, was so deafening it felt as though she was being swept along by it. Afterwards, she entertained the fans by doing a few press-ups on the track – and became the world record-holder for the number of press-ups by a female centenarian.

When I first came into contact with Ida she was 105. You would never have guessed it. Her cheeks were smooth and her neck toned, and although her frame was tiny – 4ft 6in and 5st 13lb – she held herself upright and alert. Perhaps there were hints of extreme age in her low-hanging earlobes or her gnarled, big-veined hands, or in her furrowed forehead, but in public appearances she glowed with mid-life well-being. Her voice was deep and husky, her white hair thick and curly – and her big, bright smile irresistible. 'I say my blessings every morning,' she explained.

They say that humans will endure almost anything if they feel a sense of purpose. For Ida, in later life, that purpose was fitness. She thought about it from the moment she woke up, starting with a complicated range of stretches and activation movements before even getting out of bed. 'You come into this world squirmin' and squattin' 'n' all that,' she explained, 'so why won't ya keep it up? If the babies can do it, I can do it.'

Once dressed, she would do most of her training on her exercise bike, or running backwards and forwards on her terrace, always within grabbing distance of the fence.

(Backwards and forwards meant literally that: she would alternate forward running with backward running, thus strengthening both hamstrings and quadriceps.) Then there were her exercises for strength and balance, including press-ups, and a complicated rolling 'reverse plank' routine, and squats – one-legged squats – and jumping up and down to ensure that her bones and muscles encountered resistance and impact. For the squats and the jumps, explained Shelley, 'we always have something within reach that she can grab hold of.'

Her passion for physical well-being informed everything. 'Do what you need to do, not what you want to do,' was her motto. She would always eat a big, healthy breakfast – prunes and oats were favourites – but rarely ate much in the evening. Yet she was not averse to a mid-morning shot of Hennessy cognac. She became an eloquent and irresistibly enthusiastic evangelist for the benefits of late-life exercise, especially after the publication of her 2018 memoir, *Can't Nothing Bring Me Down*, and she thrived in the media spotlight. 'Exercise is the best thing in the world,' she enthused. 'I've always been a determined person, not to let people keep me down or hold me down. But running is wonderful. Running has done great for me. It has built me up stronger than I ever was.'

Crucially, she was hardly ever still. Even when sitting down, she would move her feet restlessly, keeping all the joints and muscles activated. 'She's moving or she's asleep,' said Shelley.

Ida wasn't indestructible, though. When she was 101, she fell and fractured her right femur. Her recovery was swift: she came home with a walking frame three weeks after surgery, and within three months she was twisting on the dance floor at her 102nd birthday party – albeit with the frame within easy reach. Yet she never quite recovered her previous strength. That's the trouble with extreme old age, according to Shelley, who for many years kept a close eye on Ida's well-being in her dual capacity as daughter and coach: a single year's ageing can be transformative. 'Beyond a hundred,' said Shelley, 'the years are like dog years.'

Ida's last public race was on 25 February 2018, when she came fourth out of four runners in the Women's Open 60m in the Imperial Dade Track Classic at Armory Track & Field Center. The first three finishers were nearly 50 seconds ahead, and 102-year-old Ida, who was really just power-walking, was looking fairly tired in the final third. Then again, she was twice as old as the other three finishers combined. It was, as you'll have guessed, a world record: her sixth record in ten years and her last.

Her race was almost run. Yet one thing remained: Ida's salvaged life. Never again would she surrender to the apathy of despair. 'Running has raised me up,' she said. 'We get weak too fast,' she added. 'But you're the boss. Don't let the age keep you down. That's your body, you take care of it. Go ahead, just do it. You got to strengthen your own brain and mind. Put the age behind you.'

Comparable narrative arcs can be traced in the lives of a number of other long-lived runners, notably Fauja Singh, the most famous centenarian athlete of all. The British-Indian Sikh runner found solace in running in his late eighties after losing his daughter, wife and son in quick succession. He ran his first marathon at eighty-nine and his last at 101, and smiled ethereally in all of them. 'I run while talking to God,' he explained. He set a string of world records, including 5:40:03 as a ninety-two-year-old in the same Scotia Toronto Waterfront Marathon (2003) in which Ed Whitlock first broke three hours as a seventy-year-old (*Runner's World* called this 'the marathon's greatest day'); and 7:49:21 at the London Marathon when he was 101. He ran a 5km parkrun (in 56:55) at 105 and was still walking five miles a day when he was 108.

Another legend of late-life resilience, the American runner George A. Etzweiler, has often attributed his continued participation in mountain racing to his desire to honour the memory of his late wife, Mary, who died after sixty-eight years of marriage in 2010. Etzweiler, a retired engineer from State College, Pennsylvania, was a regular at the uphill-only Mount Washington Road Race until he was ninety-nine, and the last time I checked was still doing a 3.8-mile leg of the Tussey Mountainback 50 Mile Relay, even at 101. Why? Because to stop would be to give up – and might also feel like letting go of Mary.

Does the running help such runners to come to terms with their suffering? Undoubtedly. Does the suffering help with the running? That's harder to establish. Few people survive to their nineties or beyond without receiving some big body blows from life. Elena Pagu lost two husbands. Olga Kotelko outlived her oldest daughter, and all ten of her siblings. Sometimes, the suffering seems disproportionate or premature. The British M95 sprinter Dalbir Singh Deol saw both his parents killed in the Partition massacres of 1947. Yet other high-achieving late-life runners, such as US centenarian superstars Donald

Pellmann and Julia 'Hurricane' Hawkins, appear to have enjoyed mostly tranquil lives – if you don't count the periods of world war, or the eventual loss, in each case, of a cherished life-long spouse.

But running's role as an aid to coming to terms with pain and loss is more universal. Think of all those ordinary runners – tens of thousands of them – who every year explicitly link their most gruelling running challenges to the memories of dead friends or relatives. Whether it's a big city marathon or a couch potato's first 5k, or a champion ultra-runner's crazy halfway-round-the-world adventure, we say that we are running 'in memory of' so-and-so, or 'in aid of' an appropriate charity. We raise vast sums by doing so, yet the practical fund-raising is only part of it. The healing comes from the running itself: the effort, the sweat, the self-chosen pain. When life hit us with the original blow – the sickening, the dying, the unstoppable catastrophe – the essence of our agony as survivors was our helplessness. In running, however, we are doing something. We are fighting back. And if the challenge requires us to force ourselves through previously undreamt-of barriers of physical pain, so much the better.

This is sport as a way of taking back control, and it's by no means an exclusively modern phenomenon – as Roger Robinson points out. 'The ancient Mycenaean Greeks held games as funeral rites,' he explains. 'And the oldest accounts of athletic contests are all accounts of funeral games.' He identifies the funeral games in Book Twenty-three of Homer's *Iliad* as the oldest surviving written description of an organised running race – whose pretext is to help the Greeks come to terms with the loss of their comrade-in-arms, Patroclus; and whose shock winner, fittingly, is the veteran in the field, 'old Odysseus'.

But the former M50 world 10km road and cross-country champion has also written movingly (in *When Running Made History*) about his own redemptive experiences of running: in New York after 9/11, for example, or at the Boston Marathon that followed the 2013 bombing. Like me, he believes that there is, at some profound level, a visceral connection between running and mortality. Running, he believes, is as cathartic as music or poetry in helping the bereaved to come to terms with death, 'expressing grief and affirming life going on'.

Noora Ronkainen, the Finnish sport psychologist, believes that runners have a heightened awareness of what she calls their 'finitude'. 'I'm just thirty-six years old but I'm already slowing down. The peak is behind you at a very early age. It's like the symbolic death of the athlete. So we have to deal with something that typically people are not dealing with in their thirties.'

It doesn't even have to be about death. Sometimes mortality's most shocking blows fall years before the *coup de grace*. John Gilmour was half-broken by human cruelty while still in his twenties. The British adventurer Alex Flynn was a thirty-six-year-old lawyer when he was diagnosed with young-onset Parkinson's disease. Over the next thirteen years, before his death in 2021, Flynn ran, walked, climbed, cycled or kayaked the equivalent of 10 million metres – including a 250km Marathon des Sables, a 3,256-mile crossing of America, a 160-mile run in the Bavarian Alps, and a seven-and-a-half-day indoor 'vertical marathon' during the first UK coronavirus lockdown that involved 3,516 ascents of the stairs in his home in Wantage, Oxfordshire. Why? Partly to raise more than £1 million for Parkinson's research. But also because he was determined to be a hero. Life couldn't take that from him.

No one is immune to the damage, but the remedy is available to almost everyone. My friend David Heeley was a teenager when incipient blindness extinguished his hopes of becoming an elite middle-distance runner, so he spent the next forty years raising hundreds of thousands of pounds for charity, through extreme running challenges such as running seven marathons, on seven different continents, in seven days. Even the great Nicky Spinks, the toughest ultra-endurance athlete of her generation, began her streak of long-distance mountain record-breaking in the aftermath of a bruising brush with cancer.

You could argue that all such activities are futile. Our athletic efforts make not the slightest difference to our powerlessness in the face of mortality and decay. But they are better than doing nothing. Your chances of being on the receiving end of life's cruelties increase with each year, but courage never stops being the best response. And running never stops being a natural and effective way of focusing that courage, just as long as your legs will carry you.

23

Yes is more

In the small industrial city of Świdnica, in south-west Poland, I met a runner who was fifty years older than me. He didn't seem too bothered about sports science, or training programmes, or any of the other technicalities of running. He just ran when the mood took him, while enjoying his modest celebrity as the world's oldest competitive track-and-field athlete.

His name was Stanisław Kowalski, and I visited him on the eve of his 110th birthday, in a small apartment – in a grey, Communist-era tower block – which he shared with his eighty-one-year-old daughter, Regina. Already, he was Poland's oldest man – the oldest ever – and he was closing in on the title of Europe's oldest man. But I wanted to talk to him about his life as a sprinter.

He wasn't doing much of it by then: just occasional bursts during his daily excursions to the cemetery, where his late wife, Władysława, had been waiting for him in an elaborate double grave for a decade and a half. But it was only a few years since he had been setting world records. The last few were in the M105 category, which was created specially for him. The discus and shot put records were of debatable value: all he had to do was pick the things up and lob them a few yards in front of him. But his 100-metre record of 34.50 seconds was a serious effort: the celebrated Japanese centenarian sprinter Hide-kichi Miyazaki – 'the Golden Bolt' – was nearly eight seconds slower when he joined Kowalski in that age category a few weeks later. Come to think of it, I know people in their sixties who would struggle to run 100 metres in less than 35 seconds.

The small, bony man who greeted me was neatly dressed, with dark eyebrows, a thick head of white hair and a ready smile in which not many teeth were visible. My first thought on meeting him was that he could not possibly be as old as he said. His handshake was too firm, his cheeks were too smooth, his brown eyes too clear. Only the bony, birdlike physique suggested great age: when I looked closely, I realised that his muscles had shrunk away, so that it was his kneecaps and sternum that were pressing against his clothes, rather than his thighs and pectoral muscles. He had, said Regina, lost a lot of bulk in recent years.

If he still glowed with well-being, it must have owed much to her tireless care. She cooked for him, cleaned for him, kept an eye on him and tried, with limited success, to keep him out of mischief. Stanislaw enjoyed her solicitude with the truculent entitlement of a pampered teenager. Regina was barred from his room. He expected every meal to be just as he liked it. ('I won't eat leftovers,' he boasted. 'Vegetables should be freshly out of the ground that day.') When he went out, as he did most days, he just went. He wouldn't take a stick, despite Regina's urgings. Nor would he say where he was going or when he would be back.

She had learnt to tolerate his ways; or, at least, she had

given up hope of changing them. In any case, she knew where to look for him. Nine times out of ten, when he was out, he would be visiting Władysława in the cemetery. They had been married for seventy years, and he had yet to get over the loss. 'It's as though my heart had been taken away from me,' he told me, clutching my arm. 'She was a lovely woman. A good, quiet, elegant woman. A nice woman to kiss. I miss her.'

He had already had his name and birth date added to their shared memorial, and he visited it so regularly that, if he didn't, other frequent mourners would check the stone, to see if his missing date of death had been added. The municipal cemetery is about a mile-and-a-half from Regina's flat, and a mile-and-a-half back. He did the journey on foot. It had mostly been walking, recently, but sometimes, still, he would run.

I had been hoping to persuade him to do some running for me, but he had other plans. He was honoured by my visit, he said, and there were toasts that needed drinking. The vodka was already on the table, and we had finished our second glass by soon after 11 a.m. 'Polish vodka is very safe,' he insisted, refilling the glasses. 'It is good to have fifty grams occasionally.' 'Fifty grams' is Slavic shorthand for 'half a glass', but he was filling ours to the brim. So we talked about his memories instead.

He was born in Rogówck, a tiny village in the wooded plains of what is now central Poland, on 14 April 1910, when Edward VII was still on the British throne and Nicholas II was Tsar of Russia. The oldest of five children, Stanislaw was at different times a citizen of three different empires – Imperial Russian, Austro-Hungarian and Soviet – and he outlived them all. He had also experienced two world wars, the Great Depression, the rise and fall of Communism, and more than a century of seismic technological change. So he had learnt not to think too far beyond the day in hand, although he did share his view that, notwithstanding all the turmoils of the twenty-first century, 'the best time to be alive is today.'

His earliest memories were his worst. 'The First World War was a terrible time. I was five. The Russian soldiers came and destroyed everything.' He was talking about the Imperial Army's notorious 'scorched earth' retreat in the summer and autumn of 1915. Everything that could possibly be of use to the pursuing German forces – crops, livestock, buildings – was looted or destroyed. Civilians suffered terribly: think Russia in Ukraine in 2022. Stanislaw, with a child's eye for detail, remembered watching in agony as the soldiers ate the family's last potatoes. 'They boiled them all up, with the skins on. Then they ate them with salt.'

All five Kowalski children survived, but their parents' health was broken. Stanislaw's mother ended up having a leg amputated; his father died in 1917. Stanislaw was seven. As the eldest child, he took on a share of his widowed, disabled mother's responsibilities. As the years passed, he became the family's main breadwinner: initially in Rogówek and then, after doing his compulsory military service, in the nearby village of Brzeźnica. But jobs were scarce: this was the Great Depression. 'It was so hard, you didn't know whether to laugh or cry.' He eventually found work as a mould-maker in a cast iron foundry – a long cycle-ride away – and supplemented his meagre earnings by working on the land.

He married Władysława, who had grown up across

the street from the Kowalskis in Rogówek. His brothers
and sisters moved on. Another world war came and went.
The Nazis took some local men away to be forced labour-
ers, but Stanislaw dodged the round-up and thereafter
was left alone. 'I just worked on the land. That war didn't
make so much difference for me.'

By the time peace returned, he and Władysława had
three children. In his spare moments, Stanislaw was building a house for them all. A fourth child arrived in 1947.
Then, in 1952, just as the house was nearing completion,
Poland's new Communist rulers decided that the Kowalskis had to give up the house of their modest dreams, to
make room for the expansion of a nearby military training
zone. They were relocated to a village called Krzydlina
Wielka, 200 miles to the west, where they lived for the
next twenty-seven years. Stanislaw once again grew what
food he could but also worked as a railway signalman,
near the southern city of Wrocław – where the air is now
so polluted it's a wonder anyone lives beyond forty. Occasionally he would run a little for pleasure, 'but not proper
running'. There was neither the opportunity nor the time
for competitive athletics. He was always active, though. He
cycled eight miles to work each morning and eight miles
back in the evening – 'whatever the weather'. He rarely sat
still for long – a habit that never left him.

In 1979, Stanislaw retired. He and Władysława moved
to a small apartment in Świdnica. Each had a pension,
and the children had grown up and left, so they were able
to enjoy a period of relative comfort. 'We lived in one flat
and ate from the same pot. We could have a good life.'

Stanislaw made new friends. He liked to go out drinking with them; he even frequented the local discothèque.

He was, perhaps, a less than perfect husband. 'I was a crazy man: I liked having fun. I'm too polite to say "No" to people.' Władysława was more likely to be found at home, preparing the contents of that shared pot. But they were happy, and 'She was the boss.'

In 2003, Władysława died of a stroke. She was eighty-nine: a ripe enough age. Stanislaw, ninety-three, felt like giving up. 'When your spouse dies, you have lost something priceless. If someone gives you a box of gold and jewels, it means nothing . . .' What more could life offer him? But it turned out that he had not yet finished.

He bought that double plot in the cemetery on Lukasinskiego Street, on the northern edge of town. He had their twin slabs inscribed, and he began his daily visits. He was still doing them seventeen years later. 'I go there now, while I can, because one day, no one will go.'

As the months went by, he was surprised by the benefit he seemed to derive from those brisk daily walks, three-and-a-half miles from where he then lived and three-and-a-half miles back. 'I felt good. I was satisfied. I felt like I was born again.'

He started to enjoy himself again, going out with friends. Later, he moved in with Regina. The cemetery was now barely a mile away, so he began to walk faster. One day, he saw an item on television about a runner, relatively old, who was timing himself over a fixed distance between two pylons. 'I wanted to see if I could run at the same speed.' So he found a comparable stretch of his route, and from then on, each time he passed it, he timed himself.

He was 103 – almost 104. It never occurred to him that

this should somehow disqualify him from having a go. The weeks passed. His times improved. His enthusiasm grew. He incorporated more stretches of running into his journey, including the long, straight, dusty path, more than 100m long, that cuts through the cemetery itself.

People began to notice, including, one day, Regina, who was shocked to see her 104-year-old father running in the street and timing himself. Word spread. One day, the story of Świdnica's sprinting centenarian reached the ears of Zygmunt Worsa, the deputy mayor. Worsa, once a decent athlete himself, had spent much of his life in sports administration and coaching. He decided to investigate.

'When I first asked Mr Kowalski to come and run for me in the athletics stadium, I suddenly started to worry that I was being irresponsible,' remembered Worsa. 'So I checked with his daughter. She said: "If he wants to do it, there's nothing I can do to stop him anyway."'

'So Mr Kowalski ran 100 metres, and I timed him, and I was so astonished by what I saw that I forgot to stop my stopwatch when he crossed the line.'

Worsa then arranged another run for him, with a reputable timekeeper, and on the basis of that sub-35-second 100m he introduced Stanislaw to the competitive circuit.

Kowalski ran his first 100m event in May 2014, in the athletics stadium in Wrocław. His time, 32.79, was a European record in the M100 category (although nowhere near Hidekichi Miyazaki's 2010 world record of 29.83). Seven months later, in Poland's Indoor National Veterans' Championship in Toruń, Kowalski set world records for 60 metres (19.72) and shot put (5.08 m).

He began to think about what more he might achieve, even as the ageing process pushed him towards achieving less. According to Regina, he would sometimes become frustrated at his physical limitations, just as toddlers sometimes are. 'I have to calm him down. I tell him, it simply isn't possible for you to run as fast as you did when you were younger. But he doesn't listen.'

Meanwhile, Kowalski's fame grew. In March 2015, in Toruń again, he won gold medals for 60m and for shot put, in the European Masters Athletics Indoor Championships. The following month, he had another birthday, and that summer, at the outdoor National Veterans Championship (also in Toruń), he became the first athlete ever to compete officially as a 105-year-old. That was when he set his three most recent world records.

He was a celebrity by then. Poland's president at the time, Bronisław Komorowski, awarded him the Gold Cross of Merit, Poland's highest civilian award. Some time later, the rapper 50 Cent came across some old footage of Stanislaw racing and posted it on Facebook with the comment: 'He's 104. What's your excuse?' The comment received more than 50,000 likes.

The elderly often complain that age makes them 'invisible'. Yet Stanislaw Kowalski had arguably become Świdnica's most famous inhabitant since Manfred von Richthofen, the First World War flying ace. The only thing stopping him becoming more famous still was that he hadn't competed as an M110 (another category that would have to be created just for him). He was fit enough to do so. 'Two weeks ago I ran a hundred metres in the cemetery,' he boasted. 'It took me forty seconds.' Yet his days as a track superstar appeared to be over. His achievements in 2015 made him so famous that friends, acquaintances and relatives began to suspect that someone must be getting rich from his exploits. 'People were starting to get jealous,' said Worsa, 'so his family asked me to stop taking him to race meetings.'

This meant that, if I wanted to see Stanislaw run, I needed to catch him in the cemetery – which clearly wasn't going to happen that day, as the vodka bottle gently emptied itself. Instead, using Zygmunt Worsa's phone, we watched footage of some of his old races. It was worth seeing. Even as a 104-year-old, he didn't shuffle. He lunged forward, striking the ground forcefully with his heels and focusing on the track ahead. There was a stiffness on his left side, and his right leg strayed outward slightly, but there was no mistaking the competitive intent. It was like watching a middle-aged man dashing for a bus, stiffly but with urgent determination.

Did he have a secret? He was often asked – and gave many different answers. Sometimes he would attribute his enduring fitness to his dietary preferences: fresh vegetables; onions, garlic, honey, avoiding large evening meals and, generally, eating sparingly. ('It's better to eat too little than too much.')

Sometimes he would say that he had kept healthy by steering clear of doctors: 'I don't know doctors and doctors don't know me.' Information about his physiology is, as a result, sparse.

Sometimes he would say that it was having such a big family that kept him young. (The irony that several of his descendants are doctors doesn't bother him.) Totting up his brood for my benefit, he counted three surviving children (out of four), ten grandchildren, nine great-grandchildren and four great-great-grandchildren. 'I have so many relatives around me that Death will not come near me,' he declared.

Sometimes he would attribute his well-being to his habits of physical activity. 'I have never sat still,' he said, and to prove his point showed me a photograph of him climbing a big tree, taken when he was 100. 'Every morning,' he added, 'I do some exercises I remember from the army, to wake myself up.' His routine included squats and lateral stretches, but he was cagey about the other details – and Regina was forbidden to watch.

Often he would attribute his longevity to vodka. 'For health, vodka is better than a pill, better than medicine.' And sometimes he would attribute it to a different kind of spirit, which impelled him to 'do what I want' in nearly all circumstances. 'I always say yes to everything. That's why when the mayor' – he meant Zygmunt Worsa – 'asked me to run for him, I said yes. That's my secret. Never say no.'

He had almost persuaded me – although not quite enough to stop me saying no to his offer of yet another glass of vodka. I felt guilty for going against his affirmative philosophy, but I would have felt guiltier still had our meeting degenerated, as it threatened to do, into a drinking contest. (The one thing worse than losing such a contest with a 109-year-old would be winning one.) In any case, my lift back to Wrocław was getting impatient, and Regina clearly felt that her father needed a rest.

So I said goodbye, little the wiser about the science of late-life sprinting, or about how a middle-aged plodder can turn himself into a respectably competitive international athlete – yet feeling unexpectedly enlightened about late-life challenges in general. It isn't just about spirit, liquid or otherwise. But a generous serving of spirit clearly helps.

Stanislaw Kowalski raised his glass, and as we walked back to the car his final, defiant pledge was ringing in my ears. 'I'll never stop living till I die,' he declared.

24

Maxing out

The world championships were getting near, when my new-found sense of runner's perspective came under sudden pressure.

I had been making what felt like reasonable progress, putting in as much training as I could, as intelligently as I could, while avoiding further injuries. My focus had shifted from rehabilitation to actual fitness, and my speed, strength and stamina were clearly improving. It would be nice to say that I had been sticking diligently to a carefully calibrated programme, but that wouldn't be true. I just did what I could, when I could, vaguely incorporating much of the advice I had been given. It wasn't perfect, but my lifestyle could handle it, and I was at least improving.

Long-forgotten sensations of end-of-work-out exhilaration – when you know that you have given everything you have to give, and your whole being is saturated in sweat and endorphins – had been becoming familiar again. I knew I was still way below the appropriate standard for a world championship, but I was doing the best I could, and I was getting stronger. And that's all any late-life runner can reasonably hope for.

Then I got Covid.

It felt pretty mild, but it lingered, putting me out of sporting action for nearly a month. By the time I felt well enough to resume proper training, I was weak and podgy as a toddler. Half my muscle mass appeared to have vanished, along with half my lung capacity. It was like having a slow puncture.

I told myself not to over-react. This was hardly a notable setback, in the great scheme of things. But rejecting self-pity wasn't quite the same as maintaining self-belief. All the benefits of my recent training had been wiped out, and when I timed myself I found I was slower than I had been a year or so earlier.

Never mind, I told myself. None of this matters. You're alive, you're mobile, you're able to work and you're able to run. You're lucky. And you've booked your travel to Finland in two months' time. If that's not privilege, what is?

But I struggled to put my heart and soul back into my running. The apparent futility of my efforts had sapped me of my hunger. I could live with the fact that I wasn't much good as a runner, and even with the fact that I would soon be exposing my limitations in a rather high-profile way. What I couldn't deal with was the knowledge that all the time, effort and thought I had put into my training – all that *passion* – had simply been wasted. Human beings can, as we know, endure almost anything if they have a purpose. But if that purpose turns out to have been entirely self-defeating, why bother?

I carried on going through the motions. It was too late to back out. But I was chasing my dream dutifully, not passionately. Half-heartedness became my default mode. And when I did sometimes summon the fire to force myself through the pain barrier, the same question kept coming back to discourage me. What was the point?

John Kaag doesn't do anything half-heartedly. The forty-two-year-old professor and chair of Philosophy at the University of Massachusetts, Lowell, is renowned for the intensity of his teachings on existentialism. 'Students weep in my classes,' he boasts, quoting with pride the tearful complaint: 'I used to be happy until I discovered Nietzsche.'

He's a gentle-mannered man, but he's not a big believer in comfort zones. In his own student days, he took Nietzsche so seriously that, one vacation, he spent nine weeks hiking alone in the Swiss Alps, following in the German proto-existentialist's footsteps and pondering his ideas to the brink of madness. At one point he came dangerously close to throwing himself off a cliff – which felt, briefly, like the logical conclusion of Nietzsche's no-holds-barred thinking.

So it wasn't surprising that, when Kaag started running in his early twenties, he didn't mess around. He trained. He trained harder. He ran faster and further. And the better he got, the more intensity he demanded of himself. He wasn't a world-beater, but he became good enough to win several triathlons; and as far as he was concerned there was still room for improvement.

Within a few years, a habit that had begun as his way of taking control of his young life had taken control of him, becoming an insatiable drain on his time, energy and attention. Everything else became secondary to the simple goal of meeting his training targets. With hindsight, he recognises this as a 'compulsive mania'; at the time, it just felt like something important. Sometimes he would run hard and, for a few transcendent moments, body, spirit, breath, will, movement and environment all seemed to harmonise. But the more obsessively he trained, the rarer these moments of 'flow' became. He was too focused on his goals.

The moment he finished one run, he would plan the next. If something unexpected happened, his reaction was alarm — about the possible impact on his training plans. Nothing could come between him and his running objectives. Keeping fit had become a kind of comfort blanket for him: he lacked the energy to worry about anything else.

'I don't blame running for my first divorce,' he says, 'but it didn't help.' Likewise his second. His four-year-old daughter cried when he couldn't bring himself to slow down in mid-run to give her a hug.

After turning forty, Kaag slowed down a bit, but he didn't ease off. He could still knock off 6 to 8 miles at a time at 7-minute mile pace, and most days that's what he did. And that's what he was doing on a cold February morning in 2020. He was in the university gym at Lowell, running on a treadmill while a blizzard raged outdoors. After six brisk miles, he stepped off the machine, lay down on the floor and, with a strangely pungent sweat seeping from his body, suffered an abrupt cardiac arrest. For a minute or more he was clinically dead.

He doesn't remember who 'shocked me back to life' with a 3,000-volt jolt from a defibrillator. What he does remember was that 'I was, for the first time in years, not thinking about running.'

His admirers in academia might find that hard to

believe. Handsome, charismatic, brilliantly articulate, Kaag has been a dazzling star in the American philosophical firmament for a decade and a half. Surely he must have spent most of his time thinking about his work? For his students, who despite the tears were devoted to his classes, that was the essence of his teaching: he embodied philosophy not as a dry academic discipline but as a practical, embodied response to the problems of actual living. Yet it turned out that even Kaag's philosophical passions – Nietzsche, Camus, Schopenhauer, Heidegger, William James – preoccupied him less than his obsession with meeting his training targets. 'I had,' he reflects, 'used running as a way to run away from life rather than embrace it.'

There on the gym floor, he lay 'perfectly still' and listened with curious detachment to the far-away voices of the paramedics. He had, he learnt later, experienced a near-fatal episode of ventricular tachycardia, caused by a congenital abnormality of the right coronary artery. But all he understood at the time was that, for once, he was looking reality in the face. He would not live for ever. He might not even see tomorrow. As for his past: he had run away from things he truly cared about – in his personal life, in his work – and all for the sake of what? Even if he did survive, there was no hiding from the waste. Reality was indifferent to his fitness goals. The rest was just missed opportunities.

This felt like a shock, but it shouldn't have. It was what he had been teaching for years. Hundreds of philosophy students, present and past, have Kaag to thank for their understanding of 'the Absurd' – the term popularised by French philosopher Albert Camus to express (in Kaag's words) 'the utter dissonance between the human quest for meaning in life and the silent indifference of the universe'. Camus thought that we live best when we avoid the self-deceptions that prevent us from perceiving that dissonance, and in works such as *The Myth of Sisyphus* (1942) and *The Rebel* (1951) he argued that, too often, we do the opposite. We distract ourselves from the Absurd with habits of thought that imply, falsely, that the meanings we attach to our lives are rooted in a deeper reality. Camus called this 'philosophical suicide': in effect, putting our heads in the sand. And that, Kaag now realised, was what he had been doing with his running compulsion.

'I teach Camus every semester,' Kaag wrote later, in a much-shared 2020 essay, 'How To Live With Dying', in the *American Scholar*, 'but I didn't understand him – not even close – until I nearly killed myself on that winter day.' Hovering between life and death, however: 'at that point, the Absurd makes more sense to you.'

What it means, he told me later, is that 'It doesn't matter if you want to live for ever: you won't. It doesn't matter if you want to stay fit into your eighties: you probably won't. It doesn't matter if you don't want to have a heart attack when you're forty: sometimes you will. Nature simply doesn't care.'

This isn't, in itself, a brilliantly original insight. That doesn't stop it being true. And Kaag's experience reminds us how easy it is to combine theoretical awareness with visceral denial, or deliberate unawareness. In his case, he achieved that unawareness through running, but he could just as easily have done so through some other distraction. As he pointed out in his essay for the *American Scholar*, the modern world is awash with forces and systems that seduce us with their claims to possess 'some sort of magical, transcendent meaning': consumerism, entertainment, social media, political or religious dogma. We cling unthinkingly to the aspirations they imply: 'If I can just bank the right number of miles, if I can just get the right grades, if I can just marry the right person – my world will not go to pieces.'

But those promises are lies. Everyone's world will go to pieces, eventually, and life in the meantime is just 'the futile process of not dying'. This is a frightening and depressing thought. But the risk, for those who cling to their distracting illusions and compulsions in order to avoid thinking it, is that 'you might get to the end of your life and discover that you haven't really lived.'

Looking back on his heart attack today, Kaag considers himself fortunate: not because he survived – for a while – his unscheduled close encounter with death, but because that encounter forced him to look life in the face. Previously, he had used running as 'my distraction, my escape, my solution – the way that I tried to order a chaotic universe.' But the universe had refused to be ordered, as it always does; and Kaag was left staring at the harsh existential truths with which he had been upsetting his students for years.

That wasn't the end of his story. Forced to face up to his mortality, he realised there were better ways of living and running. He understood that 'I had been sacrificing large parts of my life' in pursuit of goals that he didn't even particularly care about. His relentless 'running away' had helped him to 'avoid certain things that I was afraid of in my personal life', but it had also blinded him to the fact that 'life can be spent doing something other than trailing your obsession.' So he has been trying, ever since, to live with more 'existential urgency'; and it seems, so far, to be working.

If you talk to Kaag today, it's hard not to be struck by the thought that, for someone whose long-cherished sporting dreams have been shattered by a catastrophic physical breakdown, he seems remarkably cheerful. But that, he says, is the point. He has had to grow: as a person and as a runner.

He had bypass surgery, and within six weeks he was running again, albeit with radically adjusted aspirations. 'When I did my first jog,' he remembers, 'I made it for half a mile. It took me eight minutes. At the end of it I cried. It was so demoralising. My wife said, "Can't you just be happy for the fact that you're not dead?"' He thought about it, and tried.

He's still trying. When I last spoke to him, Kaag was back to running 5 or 6 miles at a time, sometimes – when he felt good – at 8-minute mile pace. By the time you read this, perhaps he'll be faster. He hopes so: he still has aspirations as a runner. But there is, he insists, a difference these days: he tries not to let his training aspirations distract him from the underlying absurdity – in the philosophical sense – of having such goals at all. He strives, sometimes intensely, to be the best runner he can be. But sometimes, too, he's prepared to slow down, even stop, depending on how he feels. The important thing, he believes, is to run each day from clear-eyed choice, not from fear of what would happen if you didn't.

By one measure, he is less of a runner than he used to be. By another, he is much more, because 'I am no longer running away.' Like his traumatised philosophy students, he has been forced to leave his comfort zone – and has emerged with something stronger: 'not contentment, but growth'.

He thinks of himself as an 'old athlete' now, not because he is old or frail in any sense that I would recognise, but because he runs with a sense of his own mortality: 'We're worm-food. We are all heading for cardiac arrest. Our hearts will stop.'

He still enjoys, sometimes, the glow of self-worth that comes from a good, fast run; and he still aspires to those elusive moments of 'flow', in which the runner simultaneously loses himself and finds himself. But he tries hard to resist drifting back into his old obsessive ways, reminding himself that 'it's possible I don't have many days left' and that his life remains 'precious, fragile and ephemeral' irrespective of his self-imposed goals. 'I used to say to myself: "I have to go and train now." But you don't *have* to do anything. All you have to do is die. Running is a choice. The question is, how do you take up that choice?'

Do thoughts like this have any relevance to those of us who are *not* studying philosophy, or who do not share Kaag's bleak existentialism? I think they do, simply because, as older runners, we are by definition running out of time. Mortality is not an academic abstraction. It's the central fact of every human life. And the older you get, the bigger the shadow it casts. It's futile to pretend it isn't there – especially when you can sense your body's natural inclination to decay.

That's not to suggest there's anything foolish about setting ourselves long-term training targets and performance goals, or about turning ourselves into semi-automatons in order to achieve them. 'It's fine to make plans,' says

Kaag, 'just as long as it's a choice. If that's how you really want to spend your time, fine.' Even mindless compulsions have their place in a wisely lived life, if you choose them clear-sightedly. I clean my teeth twice a day, unthinkingly, and feel uncomfortable if I don't. I'll still end up as worm-food, but, in the meantime, my days are rarely dominated by dental problems, which feels like a good exchange for those short periods of auto-pilot brushing. Similarly, my unthinking compulsion to take some form of exercise every day – because I feel uncomfortable if I don't – feels like quite a good use of a small proportion of my time, given the obvious effects on my day-to-day health and well-being. What matters is to avoid living our whole lives on auto-pilot, and to live instead with what Kaag calls 'existential urgency'.

The trick for runners, I think, is to adapt a saying variously attributed to Desiderius Erasmus, Mahatma Gandhi and the Prophet Muhammad: 'Work as if you were going to live for ever, but live as if you were going to die tomorrow.' The wisest late-life runners train and compete with a profound, methodical commitment that appears to pay no heed to the inevitability of decay and oblivion. But they are also keenly aware that they are living on borrowed time. Every day, they feel the gravitational pull of ageing, dragging them down towards decrepitude and death. So they seize each sporting opportunity as if it might be their last.

And from that perspective, argues Kaag, it's not the older people in running who should be pitied: it's the younger ones. Young athletes are the ones who reach the end of life-defining careers of sporting glory – then reel at the bleak meaninglessness of lives in which that kind of glory is no longer an option. For older runners, failure, disappointment and obscurity are priced in. If we none the less persist, it's because we've found reasons to run that *mean* something.

And when we run to the utmost limits of our abilities, knowing that our time is running out and that nothing we will achieve as runners is of any lasting significance, we experience our sport in a richer, more glorious way than the elite twenty-somethings who bang out Olympic-level times almost routinely, simply because that's what they've programmed themselves to do. Our age-related weakness is our privilege.

No one welcomes it when Death forces his way into the foreground of our consciousness. But at least these intrusions remind us why we want to live. Young runners run faster, but they often do so unthinkingly. Those of us who choose to keep going when our bodies have begun to fail us can, if we remember, luxuriate in the experience, with all its many layers of pleasure and pain. We can, as Kaag puts it, 'own it' – seizing our moments greedily, knowing that there may not be many more; and the obvious objective futility of our endeavours diminishes neither them nor us.

I think this may be what Kaag has in mind when he says – quoting an older running buddy – that 'running is an old man's sport'. Since he realised how frail his own health was, he has been paying a lot more attention to the older runners he meets out on his local trails, and he has been struck by their ability 'to persist and endure'. Long-distance running, he believes, 'is about patience, and being long-suffering. And I think older individuals, and people who've been through some sickness, get that, in a

way that young and healthy people don't. If you've suffered through something, well, that is what we do in life.'

Kaag adds that, since self-identifying as an older athlete, he has developed 'an even deeper sense of what
Nietzsche calls the "*amor fati*", or love of fate'. Nietzsche
developed this classical concept to propose a way of
embracing your fate so unreservedly that you would be
willing, if you could, to live your life over and over again
for ever, without changing a detail. In other words, you
love not just your life as you would like it to be, or those
aspects of your life that you find most pleasing or comforting, but everything about yourself and your life,
warts, weaknesses, smells, mistakes, failures and all –
including the accelerating decay of age. 'As an older
runner,' says Kaag, 'I think that the "*amor fati*" is a very,
very important philosophical lesson.'

But his main running role model these days is the
mythical hero of Albert Camus's best-known work, *The
Myth of Sisyphus*. In Greek mythology, Sisyphus was con-
demned to spend eternity pushing a boulder up a hill,
the catch being that each time he is on the point of reaching the top, the boulder rolls back down again. For
Camus, this myth embodies the absurdity of the human
condition. 'Sisyphus has a purpose,' explains Kaag, 'but
the universe doesn't give a damn. Gravity will continu-
ally thwart him.'

But Sisyphus can also be seen as embodying the possibility of an approach to life that Camus identifies as 'revolt'.
'This is not resignation,' writes Kaag in 'How To Live With
Dying,' 'and it's certainly not denial. It is the refusal to run
away. It's the willingness to push the boulder of life with
full knowledge that one is going to eventually fail.' And

this, Kaag believes, has a special relevance for ageing runners.

'Socrates famously said that philosophy is a preparation for death, and running, I think, is somewhat similar. Running is a good way of simulating how you are going to respond to the inevitable decline of being human. You can feel that you are on the way to the final finish line, and as you get older, you realise that your body is slowly disintegrating. You wake up in the morning and your joints are sore, or arthritis sets in. One needs to adjust one's expectations to those facts of life; and as an athlete it's very difficult to do so.' But Camus, he believes, has good advice for us. 'Camus tells us to live without hope.'

He pauses, as if he were waiting for me to start crying. Students sometimes do, around this point. But I'm just thinking: yes, exactly – like the runner on the crumbling scree slope! 'Live without hope,' Kaag continues with an inclusive grin, 'and put everything you have into it anyway. Put your back into pushing the boulder. Because that's all there is. Hope is this thing that allows you to half-arse your life. But you don't want to look back on the life that you've lived and say, "Oh, that was my life? I was sleepwalking . . ." You want to say: "*That was my life!*" Whatever you do, own it.'

To clarify this idea, he likes to invoke a training routine he used to do in the gym, when you take a particular exercise and repeat it 'to failure'. Whether you do this by increasing the weight you are lifting or by continuing the repetitions indefinitely, the aim is the same: to 'max out'. You keep doing it until you can't. Eventually, there is nothing left in your muscles, and the weight won't budge. You know before you start this routine that you are going to fail. That's the point of it. But although that aspect of the process is pre-ordained, there is also an element of choice: we can choose how much of ourselves we invest in the moment. Kaag remembers one coach who used to urge him to 'leave it all on the mat' – in other words, to hold absolutely nothing back. And that is a choice each of us can make, not just as runners but in any aspect of our doomed lives that we choose to prioritise and embrace. Accept the inevitability of failure, and give it everything anyway.

According to Camus, 'We should imagine Sisyphus happy,' because 'The struggle itself towards the heights is enough to fill a man's heart.' When – in my own long-ago student days – I first came across those sentences I dismissed them as empty attitudinising. If Sisyphus was happy, he was an idiot. Who, in any case, wants to spend their days facing up to the bleakness of the human condition, when we could be distracting ourselves with deliciously comforting delusions?

Today, however, as a runner slipping down the scree slope of physiological decay, I feel the power of Camus's ideas. With each passing year, it gets harder and more pointless to deny the obvious. We are mortal. Death is waiting, and the process of dying has begun. Nothing will remain of us but dust – and perhaps a few brief ripples of love. And while it is prudent to do what we can to slow down physical decay – through planned, intelligent, forward-thinking training – a more pressing need is to shore up our defences against despair.

Once again, you don't have to be a brilliant professor to work this out. The evidence saturates our lives, and anyone who has given serious thought to the challenges of running in later life is probably thinking already in vaguely Sisyphean terms. We work harder and harder each year, for less and less reward, knowing that we'll lose in the end. The boulder is getting heavier. Our limbs are tiring. It's all uphill from here, and it will end in tears. All that is fixed. Our only choice is between surrendering now, or continuing, pointlessly, to push.

Why bother? There is no reason. 'At the end of the day, we're still just worm-food,' says Kaag. 'But what we do get to do with our time, if we choose, is to push, and to put our back into it. In other words, to invest everything we have into the moment we are engaged in.'

Most of my training runs in those days, including my speed sessions, would eventually bring me back into the village by the same route: up a rutted track that becomes a narrow, pot-holed lane, which leads in a straightish line up to my finishing-point in front of the pub. It's about 200 metres, all uphill, and regardless of what kind of session I had been doing I always felt that for that bit I ought to accelerate until my legs were burning and my lungs ready to explode. (Otherwise, what would the neighbours think?) I usually enjoyed it, though, before Covid. It wasn't too far, it wasn't impossibly steep, the finish was in sight, and I generally felt quite pleased with myself when I stopped. There was also the consolation that, for much of those 200 metres, I could distract myself with a view of the graveyard on my left: spacious, green, sloping and, for such a small and ancient village, surprisingly empty. Often, thoughts of Ed Whitlock would appear in my head, as inspiration or consolation. ('If I could keep running for as long as he did, I could have decades more of interesting, active life ahead of me . . .')

And so, sometimes, would the thought that, somewhere on Earth, there is a spot where, one day, my own remains will be laid. 'Will it be here?' I would wonder; and, while I was at it: 'I wonder if anyone will look back on my life and consider it well-lived?' More constructively, I would wonder if I myself – reaching that date in the calendar that will one day become the date on which I died – would look back on my life and consider it well-lived. Such thoughts seem morbid in print, and probably weird. But they would usually occupy my mind just enough to see me through that final half-minute or so of intense uphill effort; and, most times, they felt healthy.

But my post-Covid deflation had left me feebler mentally as well as physically, and in recent weeks my pleasure in that final run-in had dried up. None of this training seemed to be making me any fitter, and the hopelessness of my position had sapped my fighting spirit, leaving only my coward's negativity. A daunting struggle? I would never make it. Effort? It wouldn't be enough. Pain? It was too much. Even that short uphill sprint had begun to feel like an unendurable slog.

In the days following my conversation with John Kaag, however, I realised that I could think about my difficulties in a slightly more constructive way. Yes, there was plenty to despair about. I was going to fail in Finland. I was going to lose, badly and painfully. But isn't that what Masters sport means? You always lose. We can set ourselves what targets we like – records, medals, vaguely respectable times – and invest every drop of our energy and will into achieving them. But time and physiology, irrespective of the outcome, will make a mockery of it all. Every single athlete who competes in Masters, even the medallists and record-breakers, will be defeated, in the end, by age. We will grow slower and weaker, wither and die; and any traces of our sporting prowess that survive us will fade very quickly afterwards to nothing.

And there, I realised, is the ultimate beauty of late-life running. *All your striving is doomed to failure.* Once you recognise that, you are free to dream as boldly as you like. If I am going to fail anyway, why limit my ambitions? I might as well fail to win a gold medal as a bronze one. I might as well be beaten by the best runners who are prepared to race against me. I will lose, embarrassingly, but so what? In the long run, we are all losers.

And for runners like me, there is an added bonus: our limited talent. Far from being a cause for despondency, the vast gulf in ability between me and the best of my age was liberating, precisely because it was so huge. I could achieve all my most ambitious training aims, and end up running 10km 4 or 5 minutes faster than my current best, and Yoshitsugu Iwanaga's world record could be 4 or 5 minutes slower than it is, and I would still have no hope of getting near it, even with a year of elite coaching and full-time training. So why worry? Losing by a huge margin was a given. The only question was: was I ready to give it my best shot?

One June morning, with barely three weeks left before the world championship, I began that final uphill run-in, and I realised that maybe I was ready. I might not be very fit, but I was no longer ill, I had no new injuries, and, in short, I had nothing to lose. Why not go for it? In other words, I would stop worrying about what I was achieving and would focus instead on whether or not I was 'leaving it all on the mat'. And I would start now.

I lengthened my stride, drove forwards and upwards with each step, swung my arms as if they were carrying heavy weights. I was still on the muddy stretch when the oxygen ran out, but I wasn't bothered. The struggle and pain were the point. I was going to suffer because I chose to suffer: because I wanted to enjoy the sensation of striving until my legs gave out.

And I did.

I eased off in the final strides. I had to: I had run so hard I had nothing else to give. When I stopped, I bent double, almost crying with discomfort and relief. My whole body felt sick, my legs were trembling, and I felt a strong urge to groan. And then, very quickly, elation flooded my being.

Swaying happily on my rubbery legs, I staggered the remaining metres to my door, thinking of the pain and humiliation to come and resolving to try to enjoy the experience. I might not amount to much as a runner, but I had, I thought, finally understood the most beautiful secret of Masters athletics. The glory isn't in winning. It's in facing up to the inevitability of ultimate defeat.

And then doing it anyway.

25

First World problems

The gun barked. A hundred and twenty-eight runners, from thirty-one nations, sprang into action: lean, muscular, taut with focus. They had been training for this for years, and you could sense their pent-up energy as they bounded forward. This was a battle, with the gloves off, for world championship medals; and all but the toughest would finish empty-handed.

I stumbled behind them as best I could, trying to find an appropriate rhythm. The leaders were quickly hidden by the chasing pack, but I felt the pull of their wake. I could already tell that, like many people, I was running much faster than was sensible. But what was the point in coming here, if I didn't?

I did need to keep this up for 10km, though, and after barely 200 metres I was having doubts. The afternoon was oven-hot: July sun beating back on us from the tarmac. The thought of carrying on like this for a whole race made me nauseous.

Never mind, I told myself, you've done the difficult bit; and in a sense I had. I had avoided further injury, got through Covid, made it to Finland, found my way to the right city and, today, to the right Exhibition & Sports Centre on the edge of town, where the non-stadium races of the 2022 World Masters Athletics Championships were being held. I seemed to have jumped through all the necessary hoops in terms of entry, registration and pre-race procedures and had made it to the starting line at the right time, in the right national kit (Great Britain Masters, £50 for vest and shorts). I had, in fact, showed up. Now all I had to do was run.

But running is easier on some days than on others, and today, I sensed, was an 'other'. The nearest I had to a pre-race plan was a vague vision that I would distract myself by enjoying the sights of Tampere. But for the first mile or so there was almost nothing to see: just a long, carless car park with a line of small trees down the middle, alongside a straight, empty road, and what looked like a series of car dealerships fenced off beyond. Once I had taken that in, there was nothing to occupy my thoughts except running: what it felt like, what it ought to feel like, what it was going to feel like; and those eager, gifted runners ahead, powering ahead relentlessly; and a panicky sense that I was being left behind.

I tried to calm myself with thoughts of gratitude. What a huge, ridiculous, unearned privilege this was, I reminded myself, to be running here today. I thought of all the millions of people my age who couldn't possibly consider doing such a thing. I thought of all the people struggling with day-to-day life back in Britain. The least I could do was enjoy my good fortune – and make a go of it.

But gratitude doesn't make you an athlete. By the first kilometre marker I was gasping for breath; by the second (reached after doubling back on ourselves in the car park), I was hanging on for dear life. I felt sick with self-pity and regret. What had I done? All those fancy thoughts I had

had back in England about dreams and adventures seemed fatuous. I was simply out of my depth: horribly so. Yet I could hardly drop out now. I would just have to hope that, somehow, I could cling on to the end; and that the end would come soon.

The route began to climb slightly, up a biggish road. There were houses on our left, I think, but dense garden foliage made them hard to see, and in any case the rising physical discomfort had shrunk my mental horizons. I was aware of the half-dozen runners immediately ahead of me, strung out in a lengthening line; and I could hear the breathing of the runner behind me. But that was about all. I reckoned that there might be a dozen or more runners somewhere behind me, mostly from the M65 category. But I did know that there were an awful lot of runners in front, and that most were already out of sight.

There were seven male age groups in the race, from M35 to M65. The women of all ages and the seventy-or-over men would be running the same course later – although how much later might depend on how long it took me to finish. I was resigned to finishing a mile or more behind the front-runners of this younger men's race, and although I hoped not to finish absolutely last of all, I accepted that this might happen. But I really didn't fancy being overtaken by the leaders of a subsequent race, or forcing the organisers to delay its start, so I dug deep to keep my pace up.

It was getting harder. There was no breeze and little shadow: just fierce, unblinking sunlight. My legs already felt drained: from the speed, from the heat, from their lack of recent miles; and, I suspect, from the tensions of the preceding hours and days. I had, I realised, been feeling very anxious about this race for a long time: fretting about my health and fitness, about travel arrangements, about the challenge of behaving like a proper athlete in the utterly unfamiliar world of hard-core international competition. None of that mattered now. But all those neurotic weeks, at home and abroad, had squandered valuable reserves of emotional energy.

The odd thing was that in other respects my time in Tampere had been joyous. It's hard not to feel cheerful when you're sharing a small industrial city in Finland with more than 4,600 over-age athletes, from eighty-seven nations. From the moment I stepped off the train, there had been Masters on every pavement, in every café, on every tram, all glowing with physical well-being and child-like excitement. Just seeing the names on the track-suits made the world feel a warmer place: Paraguay, Jamaica, Serbia, Thailand, Mongolia, Namibia . . . Didn't they know there was a war on? Or a lingering pandemic?

The sparks of interaction were the best bits: random connections between strangers, often separated by thick barriers of language, or warm reunions between rivals from past championships. Each time I made a new acquaintance – Josef the Czech thrower, Taisto the Finnish 400m runner, Geraldine the Irish hurdler, Nageen the Indian distance runner – I felt enriched. But the sporting action had been life-enhancing too, and some of it had been unforgettable.

Maybe your eyes will glaze over when I tell you that Angela Copson, who had spent much of 2021 struggling with health problems, won emphatic golds in the W75 800m, 1500m and 5,000m (with a fourth expected to follow today in the 10km road race) and set two world records (3:07.19 for 800m and 22:53.55 for 5,000m). If so, unglaze them. Those who watched these extraordinary runs knew they were seeing sporting history made. Likewise those who saw Alastair Walker, the Scottish world record-holder, winning the M65 5,000m by half a lap, with a time (16:43.44) that would also have won him medals at M50 and M55; or Jane Horder (one of eight British hurdlers to win gold) setting a world record winning the W65 300m hurdles in 52.33 seconds; or Germany's Hartmut Krämer winning the M80 100 metres in 14.31 seconds, with seven other flat-out octogenarians within a second and a half of his world record time; or ninety-four-year-old Bhagwani Devi Dagar, from India, winning the W90 100 metres in 24.74 seconds (just under six-and-a-half-minute mile pace); or David Carr, from Australia, winning the M90 steeplechase (2,000m, eighteen hurdles, five water jumps) in 12:50.43.

Best of all, perhaps, had been the French superstar Nicole Alexis, sixty-two, winning the W60 100m and 200m with world record times (13.20 seconds and 27.78 seconds respectively) that wouldn't have been the slowest for those distances had she run them at the 2021 Tokyo Olympics. And these, of course, are just a handful of highlights, from a fortnight-long festival in which literally thousands of people demonstrated, delightedly, that being 'the wrong side' of a particular age was no barrier to being vigorously and sometimes spectacularly active.

I felt privileged to have witnessed so much rarefied sporting genius. Yet I didn't feel very empowered by it: not right now. If anything, I felt the opposite. The medallists and record-breakers showed what proper, serious, world-class Masters athletes could achieve, and it was brutally clear now that not one of those adjectives applied to me. In which case – well, it hardly needed saying. I was in the wrong place. And over the next four or five miles that was going to become increasingly, painfully and embarrassingly obvious.

I tried not to think about the next kilometre marker but kept looking for it anyway. My attempts at positive thinking had dissolved into bitter regret. How could I have been so stupid and arrogant? Why hadn't I focused on reaching world championship standard first, rather than simply signing up to compete? A proper athlete could be drinking in the excitement of a race like this, but all I could think about was that I already wanted this to be over – and that it was nowhere near over. Strange, I reflected, to come all the way to Finland just to experience a feeling like that. And strange, too, how whole years of your life can drift past almost unnoticed, yet even five minutes of running on the threshold of pain can seem to last for ever.

Which reminded me: I needed a mind trick or two, to distract me from the pain. So I tried to recite in my head all the scraps of Finnish I had learnt since arriving in Tampere. This provided excellent distraction, but I ran out of scraps very quickly. Then I attempted to repeat the flight of fancy I had used at that 10,000m race in Wimbledon, when I visualised distance run as years lived. It didn't really take off this time. My progress between kilometres seemed far too slow to make the fantasy interesting. Then I thought: OK, I'm going to retrieve a significant memory from each year of my adult life. That should pass some time.

I was somewhere between the 2km and 3km markers at this point, so metaphorically I was in my mid-twenties.

If I conjured up a specific, vivid memory for each year from the age of twenty-five onwards, and savoured and pondered the details, with a bit of luck I would have passed 3km before I got into my metaphorical thirties; at which point I could repeat the process for that decade too, and so on. Ten years per kilometre, filling my mind with emotionally rich recollections all the way up to just after the 6km marker. After that I would need a new trick, but by then more than half of the race would be behind me.

This exercise worked slightly better, but not much. I just couldn't come up with enough vivid memories. My mind was awash with vague, jumbled ones: broadly similar events and experiences that had more or less merged into one another. But substantial, exciting moments I could confidently link to a specific time and place? Alarmingly elusive.

The reason soon dawned: my past itself had been a lot more blurred, much of the time, than my current self would like it to have been. In my twenties, it had been a blur of fecklessness, drunkenness, debt and failure, in which parties, hangovers and shambolic relationships blended interchangeably. My thirties had been over-dominated by running: thousands of near-identical hours of obsessive, repetitive training, with equally fungible hours of nappy-changing as the main variation. In my forties and fifties, it was work, work, work, randomly complicated by domestic responsibilities and the competing needs of growing children and elderly parents. Then came my sixties, and the lockdown years.

I suppose many lives are like that: always busy, always short of time, always rushing to the next thing – and rarely if ever breaking tried-and-tested routines, let alone pausing to dwell in the moment. Perhaps that isn't such a bad way to live. At least it gets things done. But one of those things is life itself. Most of my time on earth was behind me now, and I wasn't sure that a mere blur was what I really wanted from whatever years remained.

So I made a resolution, soon after the 4km marker, where the course curved into a slightly quieter street. From now on, I decided, I would make a conscious effort to live in the here-and-now as much as possible, and this race seemed like a good place to start. If I was lucky enough to have such experiences as this, I shouldn't blot them out to make them manageable. I should soak up every detail gratefully. For a while, therefore, that's what I tried to do, focusing on every positive I could think of. I was running in a world championship race, in Finland, at the age of sixty-two. I was going quite fast – hence the pain. Perhaps, if I chose, I could go faster. I was in a strange, beguiling city, within a few hundred miles of the Arctic Circle, among gifted runners from all over the world. How could I possibly not feel delight, or at least excitement?

The more I thought about this, the more it reminded me that, even within the already fortunate world of Masters athletes, I was one of the luckier ones. Plenty of better and more dedicated athletes than me hadn't made it to their starting lines in Finland. In some cases, the reasons were poignant: Tony Bowman was no longer well enough to travel; neither was Eleanor Pagu. Others, such as Tommy Hughes and Gene Dykes, had pulled out because of injury. Earl Fee, discouraged by a combination of distance, a sore leg and the fact that 'It's hard to win medals when you're at the top of your age group', had reluctantly decided against the long journey; as had Alan Carter (whose hopes of being allowed to compete as an eighty-five-year-old had come to nothing); and Charles Allie, who, in addition to being at the very top of his age group, was still rebuilding his fitness after being treated earlier in the year for prostate cancer. And then there were those whose luck ran out after reaching Tampere, such as Steve Peters and Virginia Mitchell, both forced to withdraw from their 400m events (although Peters had at least won gold in the M65 100m and 200m by then). Everyone's luck runs out at some point; mine, for some reason, hadn't.

This pep talk produced enough pep to put a spring in my step for a hundred metres, maybe two. But positive thoughts fade quickly when you're running. You go faster for a while, but then, as a result, the discomfort builds, making it harder to think about anything beyond a single narrow objective: to keep going until it's done. And that, in effect, means negative thinking: longing for it all to be over; blocking out the pain of the here-and-now until you barely notice anything.

Now I was confused. Should I dwell in the sensations of the moment or prioritise grim survival? I compromised by focusing on my surroundings. The bright northern sunlight; the little detached houses with their red roofs and leafy barriers of trees and hedges – none of which, mysteriously, seemed to cast any shadow. Who lived here? And what did the inhabitants of this sleepy street feel about having thousands of over-aged athletes descend on their city? It occurred to me that most people in the world might see this spectacle rather differently than we athletes did. By normal standards, the entire championship was a festival of late-life self-indulgence.

Even the world record-breakers were, as Steve Peters put it, 'just elderly people having fun'; the rest of us couldn't even claim to be redefining the boundaries of physical possibility. We were simply in it for ourselves: a few thousand lucky members of some of history's most privileged generations, largely drawn from the world's more affluent societies, playing at being elite athletes in our replica national kit.

Even as I thought this, however, I realised that I didn't believe it. Yes, we were privileged and self-indulgent, and often shamefully self-obsessed. Our injuries and embarrassments and other insecurities could quite reasonably be dismissed as 'First World problems'. Yet that was only half the story. The simplest definition of a First World society is one that produces unfeasibly large numbers of old people, and for most such societies each old person is a problem: a burden, needing support. But Masters have taken it upon themselves to turn back the physiological clock, through competitive sporting activity; and, as a result, need less support. We make ourselves ridiculous by pursuing our childish, selfish pleasures, but we also rescue ourselves from isolation, insularity, lack of purpose and, for a while, the age-related erosion of our physical independence. Would it really help anyone if we didn't do this, but sat at home instead: couch-bound First World problems for someone else to solve?

In any case, I reminded myself, it really didn't matter what anyone else thought. That was one of the most important lessons I had ever learnt about late-life running. If you want to do it, you just have to do it. Other people can think what they like.

You do, however, have to run, and I hadn't even reached

the halfway stage yet. How could time be passing so *slowly*?

Then I saw the runner in front of me cheating.

Some small red cones showed where our route went round the bend, and he cut the corner. He can barely have shaved a second off his time, and it must have occurred to him that the person behind would see. Yet he did it anyway.

I couldn't work up any righteous anger. He had gained a metre or two, but it couldn't affect the result in any way that mattered. Neither of us would be going home with a medal. What I did feel, however, was a strange surge in morale. So I wasn't the biggest loser in the race. I would at least go home knowing I had run 10km at a world championship. He would be stuck with the knowledge that he had run only 9.999km.

A little later, I overtook him, and then, as happens when you overtake, felt obliged to press on, for fear of an embarrassing counter-attack. By the time I reached the safety of the next bend, an unnerving burning sensation was gripping my thighs and calves. I tried to ignore it, just as I tried not to agonise about where the next kilo-metre marker had got to. (Had I missed it?) Focus on your movements, I told myself. Was I using my 'spinal engine'? Were my toes relaxed? Was I lifting my knees? Were my ankles bending properly – or as close to prop-erly as they could? I think the answer to most of these questions was 'no', but it helped to ask them.

We were now in a long, straight, flat, residential street. I think it was called Perkiönkatu, but for all I could see of the houses behind the hedges it could have been any-where. There did seem to be a kilometre marker in the distance, but I searched in vain for shadows, or even a bend in the road. My world had narrowed to one grey stretch of narrow, threadbare, iron-hard tarmac. It appeared to go on for ever.

I realised that I no longer really cared where I finished or what my time would be. I just wanted to survive. Yet I also dimly remembered that, earlier on, I had cared quite a lot about what I could make myself do in this race. So I tried again to crowd out my feebleness and self-pity with more positive thoughts, this time about some of the notable Masters who had run this distance before me: far older runners who would never have dreamed of stopping, or even slowing down, when the going got tough. I thought about Ken Jones and Ginette Bedard; about Denise LeClerc and Yoko Nakono. I thought about Angela Copson, warming up at that very moment for her own attack on this course, in which she hoped (with good reason) to claim her fourth W75 gold of the championships. And I thought, too, about John Gilmour and Ed Whitlock, decades older than me when they ran their last distance races but still, somehow, unbreakable. 'Get up, Gilmour,' I said to myself. 'In no way is running in a race going to defeat you.'

The 5km marker came and went, and I found myself remembering footage I had seen of Yoko Nakono in mid-race: the neat, careful steps, the tidy arms, the smiling face. Of course. 'Enjoy yourself,' she told me. 'If you enjoy yourself, you'll go faster.'

So I put a smile on my face. '*Smile, smile, smile,*' I chanted in my head, in rhythm with my breathing. 'Be grateful,' I added. In fact, I had even more to be thankful for now, because I had survived the first half of the race and had barely three miles to go. 'Enjoy yourself, damn it!'

But the heat was worse than ever, my mouth was dry, my chest felt tight, my stomach felt simultaneously bloated and queasy, the nearest runners were fifty metres ahead, and my knees and feet were aching from the relentless pounding. All I could do was try to block out the pain until it was over.

So I thought about my running hero, Emil Zátopek, and the miraculous Olympic weeks he had spent in Finland, winning three distance-running golds in eight magical July days, exactly seventy years earlier. His third gold, in the marathon, had been his first ever attempt at the distance, yet somehow he had found the self-belief to keep pushing the pace, on endless, flat, straight Finnish roads – roads much like these – all the way to an Olympic record. 'If you can't keep going, go faster,' was Zátopek's motto. Very well: I forced myself to accelerate.

My stride may have lengthened. The gap between me and the group ahead may have narrowed a little. But it didn't last. By the 6km marker I just wanted to be sick, or failing that to lie down, and there was no question of going anything but slower. It was a shame, but it was a fact. I hadn't even covered 4 miles yet, but I was running on empty.

We had, I think, emerged from Perkiönkatu by now and, after a few more wiggles, were running along the side of a busy main road, which curved rather steeply uphill. Somewhere near the top, I felt, there must be a 7km marker, but I tried not to think about it, in case this was wishful thinking. Instead, I kept pushing, as hard as I could bear. Just keep going. And don't stop.

Eventually, I saw the 7km marker, but from the way

my legs felt it could have been the 23-mile marker in a marathon. The younger front-runners would be finishing by now. Even the M60s would be within sight of the end, psyching themselves up for that final race-deciding kick. All my grand fantasies about making myself proud had been washed away by the tide of nausea and exhaustion. The best I could hope for was to avoid abject humiliation. Well, that would be something. But I needed to do something about it.

In my head I began to yell at myself. This was the world championship! I was representing my country! The least I could do was grit my teeth through another fifteen minutes of non-lethal agony.

But another voice in my head (the sensible one) had a different view. What was the point? I was clearly going to finish the race, somehow; close to the back but probably not last of all. Everything else was detail: a few seconds here or there – maybe even a few minutes here or there – would make no difference to anyone, not even me. In which case, why suffer?

I realised I could simply slow down to a more tolerable pace. No one will know, I told myself. No one will care. You can go as slowly or as fast as you like.

Then I thought: isn't that the story of all our lives? We chase our dreams, load up our lives with status and achievements and illusory security, strive and fight with every ounce of our strength and courage – but in the long run it all vanishes. Maybe for a moment we can cause a stir, in our own hearts or in someone else's, and maybe a remembered trace or two of our time on earth will live on after us in the lives we touched. But not for long.

Within two generations – three at most – even that will be gone. Your most passionate strivings will be lost and gone. *No one will know. No one will care.*

And at that point I forgot the discomfort of running too fast. Maybe it helped that the gradient was now slightly downhill. But mainly I was pre-occupied by a fierce, angry resentment of mortality. Damn it, did life really have to be that fragile and ephemeral? Heartbreaking memories flooded my mind: of loved ones I had already lost. I could feel both their presence and their absence: family, friends, neighbours, colleagues and – while I was at it – any number of public figures whose faces had once towered over my mental landscape like US presidents on Mount Rushmore. It wasn't the prospect of my own dying that bothered me. It was the feeling that my world was predeceasing me. All that permanence, all those shared memories and values, all gone. And this was just a foretaste of what was to come.

If I hadn't been running, I think the sadness might have overwhelmed me. Instead, the action of pounding my legs on the tarmac, and the option of pounding harder, helped me reclaim a sense of being vigorously alive. It hurt. I could make it hurt more. So I wasn't entirely helpless. And if I could force my body to subject itself to this, my life's story hadn't vanished. Not yet.

I was still thinking about life's tragic transience when I realised I could see both the Exhibition & Sport Centre and what must have been the 8km marker. Hope flooded into my veins. We still had to do another long loop of the car park, but I had a clear view now of what still had to be done. And I knew that, somehow, I could do it.

Parts of the route were lined with spectators. Some

looked like runners who had already finished. It was still a welcome distraction. 'Great run, Richard,' shouted an English voice I vaguely recognised from earlier. (Thank you, whoever that was.) 'Now let's have a strong finish.'

That's easy for you to say, I muttered to myself. I was thinking more of plodding on pluckily. But then I thought, sod it: am I going to do my best or not?

So I set off in vaguely aggressive pursuit of the runner in front, twenty or thirty metres ahead. My legs weren't keen: my hamstrings had developed a rubbery wobble, and there was a fuzzy burning sensation around my knees. But the gap gradually closed, and in due course I passed him – realising, as I did so, that he was an M65, irrelevant to my finishing position. I kept pressing forward, even so, to put a gap between us, and tried to focus on the next runner, far, far ahead.

There really was no prospect of catching up this time, with barely 1,200 metres left, and in any case my calves were starting to cramp. But I kept up the painful rhythm as much as I could, gritting my teeth in the knowledge that it had to stop soon – didn't it? In any case, what was the worst that could happen? Death? Somehow that didn't bother me much, apart from the effect it would have on my finishing time. What I really didn't want was to feel that I hadn't done my best.

So I kept my eyes on the reddish vest of the runner up ahead. Just keep pushing. Or rather, keep pulling: hauling yourself towards the target ahead. Some kind of metaphor for the human condition, probably, but my brain was now too scrambled for rational thought.

Barely 600 metres remaining. The gap hadn't closed at all. There was nothing left I could do – short of stopping – that would affect my finishing position. None the less, I chose to keep trying, because . . . well, I didn't really know why. Not any more. Except that, in spite of everything, I wanted to.

Somehow I had to go faster. I thought about smiling, and about moving freely, like the breathtakingly fluid middle-aged 400 metre runners I had been watching in the stadium earlier in the week. I lifted my knees (or that's how it felt) and stretched out my stride (ditto), and imagined my hair flowing behind me, like Alan Carter's, or perhaps even bouncing in a ponytail like Jo Pavey's. Run like a happy child, I told myself.

It made little difference. By the time I emerged from the course's final wiggle to see the FINISH sign directly ahead, the red-vested runner was disappearing past it. He too had been doing his best. But I still tried to sprint the final 50 metres, imagining myself on a scree slope, driving furiously upwards until my muscles failed completely. And as I did so, a strange thought occurred to me: I didn't feel old at all. Knackered, yes, and parched and foot-sore and knee-sore and desperate to stop. But age? I had no sense of it. I was exactly the same so-so runner I had always been: not very fast, not very graceful, prone to eccentric mid-race musings and late-race self-pity but generally hardy enough to keep going to the end. And although this wasn't anything to be proud of, it did, briefly, feel like something to be very glad about.

My attempted sprint must have looked like a drunken stagger. In my head, however, I was running freely: uninhibited, for once, by middle-aged fear. And when I crossed the line, simultaneously stepping into the delicious cool of the hangar-like sports hall, I was engulfed by waves of the kind of vast, unqualified, omni-sensory happiness that is usually experienced only by children.

I can barely describe what happened next. The euphoria was too rich, too dizzying. I could stop, sit down, drink, rest, luxuriate in the fact that the ordeal was over. I could share my luminous joy with a whole crowd of other runners who had just had broadly the same experience. The red-vested runner and I embraced, congratulating one another and reproaching one another for running too fast. He was a short, stocky Puerto Rican, called Harry, who looked much younger than me and was (I think) competing in a world championship for the first time; my delight in the moment felt all the richer for being shared with him. The feeling appeared to be mutual. He smiled infectiously, and insisted on endless photos of the two of us together, and I realised with startling certainty that if we ever meet again we will meet as friends – because who else could ever really understand our near-identical ordeal on the roads of Tampere?

An electronic monitor revealed that I had come nineteenth out of twenty-three M60 finishers – a lot better than I had feared. My time, if you're interested, was 45:41, which is respectable for a middle-aged recreational runner but barely jogging pace for a proper world title contender. (It was, however, 2 minutes faster than I had run at the Northampton 10k five weeks earlier, and about 6 minutes faster than I had been managing a couple of years before that, when I first thought about trying to haul myself out of my mid-life running slump.) Eight runners in our age group went under 40 minutes, with nine more under 45; then came Harry, with me 8 seconds behind. Of the two other British M60s, Steven Doxey came fifteenth, in 43:44, while Stephen Watmough, with a seriously fast 36:38, missed out on a bronze by 9 seconds. The winner, Francisco García of Spain, beat me by over ten minutes, in 35:13.

But even he would have been well beaten by Britain's Alastair Walker, whose winning time in the M65 category, 34:44, was just outside the M65 world record (34:32) he had set in Grangemouth three months earlier. Walker's nearest challenger at M65 was more than 5 minutes slower, and he was faster than the M55 winner, too, so it wasn't just me that felt completely out of his league. Given that he used to be a 66-minute half-marathon runner (he quit the sport at thirty-eight but resumed at fifty-eight); and that he usually runs about 70 miles a week, including two intense sessions of intervals or speed-work; and that he doesn't appear to be carrying an ounce of superfluous body fat – I was lucky to finish as close to him as I did. At least I can now say I once raced against him.

As for my own performance, it turned out that I could have run a whole minute slower without it affecting my finishing position. Much of my self-inflicted suffering had, in that sense, been totally unnecessary. Yet it didn't in any way feel wasted. I had done my best – and that minute's worth of extra effort may well have been the best thing about it.

And then . . . but you don't need to know much more. We hung around, we chatted, we took more pictures and promised to share them later. We moaned happily about the toughness of the race and shared our guilty delight that it was the women and the over-seventies, not us, whose road-race was just beginning.

Most of us found our way back to the main stadium, eventually, at Ratina, in the city centre. Some of us subsequently ate, queasily in my case. And then, just as I was about to retreat to my edge-of-town Airbnb, I wandered down on a whim to Eteläpuiston, a park behind the stadium that overlooks the southernmost of Tampere's two great lakes.

It was getting on for 10 p.m. by then – I don't know where all the hours had gone – but it wasn't yet dark, and I had realised that I risked leaving Finland without having seen a lake. So I picked my way down among water birches and Norway maples to the lakeside, then sat for a long time on a log, enjoying the stillness of the water. This was Pyhäjärvi, I think: the holy lake. It seemed in those moments the most peaceful place in the world.

The opposite shore was distant and dense with trees, from which thin factory chimneys rose at irregular intervals, along with a single church tower. Far from land, a ferry appeared to be drifting, noiselessly, across the shining water, inching towards Tampere. I felt too happy to move. Then, from nowhere, a pair of heavy waves – presumably the ferry's wake – slapped clumsily on the muddy shore. A fierce storm of mosquitoes burst from the disturbed shallows, at which point I fled.

Suddenly weary, I found my way back to the city centre, cursing the mosquito that had bitten me on the neck and, for some reason, reflecting neurotically on today's race. Could I really not have gone 8 seconds faster, if I'd been a bit braver in the middle of the race, and thus claimed eighteenth place? In fact, shouldn't I have gone under 45 minutes? (Races always seem easier when you're no longer running them.) Then I thought: *what's wrong with you?* Can you really not relax for a moment and take pleasure in what has happened? You've gone from being a washed-up almost-ex-runner to being a proper Masters athlete. You're sixty-two, you've spent the past week enjoying athletics with a crowd of kindred spirits you'd never even met before, from all over the world, and you've just come nineteenth in a world championship. Just be grateful and enjoy it.

So I was and I did. But I also thought – because this is how runners' minds work – about how I might improve in future. It would be nice to get a little closer to world championship standard, even if I couldn't justify the extravagance of another trip like this. Perhaps, with a year or two of serious, intelligent training, I could bring down my time by several minutes; and in the meantime, of course, the threshold for being good for my age would come back to meet me. If I started work on it now, I could be a much better M65 than I am an M60.

I think this is an example of what should be known as the Masters Fallacy, in which you forget not just the risks of injury and further age-related decline but the fact that your current rivals are moving up through the age groups with you, making similar plans. As fallacies go, however, it's a life-enhancing one, because it faces forward. Life is always enhanced when you're contemplating your hopes for the future. I didn't even know what my goal was yet, but already I was looking forward to a better tomorrow; planning for improvement, not decline.

I reached my tram stop to find there were no trams running on the line I needed. Too sleepy to work out a public transport alternative, I set off on foot. I liked the idea of extending this post-race evening a little longer, before it vanished.

Much of the route was along a tree-lined dual carriageway. I don't remember seeing a single moving car. Tampere was asleep, which seemed odd. It was, to be fair, the middle of the night; but it barely gets dark in July when you're 150 miles north of Helsinki. There was a hint of mauve in a distant bank of clouds, and a curiously soft, milky quality to the light elsewhere. Otherwise, the only clue to the time was the dream-like silence.

I walked slowly. I didn't want the journey to end, and in any case walking fast hurt. The further I got from the city centre, the more potent the white night's magic felt. The low, square apartment blocks, concrete and pastel-painted, seemed so redolent of a previous era that I could have been in a strange, Cold War-themed science fiction movie. Seagulls screamed invisibly, oblivious to the time of day, and I noticed a scent in the air a bit like honeysuckle. Then I realised that, from the corner of a residential side street, a huge grey hare was staring out at me, eyes bulging with bewilderment.

What a strange, surprising, wonderful world it is, I reflected, and how easy it would be not to notice. But tonight I noticed, and now I understood why. In running today's race, I seemed, in a small but significant way, to have changed myself. Not only had I reawakened my inner athlete. I had reawakened my inner child: ignorantly fearless, innocently selfish, with dreams far bigger than my talents, and full of trusting hope about what might lie around the corner.

I had won neither medals nor glory. I probably never would. I was still just a slow, ageing, recreational runner. But tonight I would be dreaming in colour.

Acknowledgements

So many people have helped me with this book, at every stage of its creation, that it would be impossible to thank them all by name without making the finished product unfeasibly long. To save space: I very gratefully acknowledge the contribution of each person whose name appears in the main text of the book – many of whom shared far more of their time, experience and insight than their brief appearances might imply.

I do, however, particularly single out Neil Baxter, Angela Kikugawa, Nick Lauder, Alex Rotas and Ken Stone for special thanks, for providing encouragement, guidance and feedback beyond the call of duty.

In addition, I am grateful to the following: Samantha Amend, Lyn Atterbury, Jeff Battista, Ken Bedard, John Bridger, Ugo Carraro, Amélie Clement-Flet, Denis Daly, Carol Dickinson, Anne Dockery, Morgan Dun-Campbell, Adharanand Finn, Giuseppe Gambino, Andrew Haig, Charles, Sarah and Richard Hill, Mahmut Hilmi, George A. Hirsch, Archie Jenkins, Eileen Jones, Shelley Keeling, Beat Knechtle, Anna Kudrnová, Brett Larner and Mika Tokariarin, Mal McCausland, Anna Misiak-Terenkoczy, Tony Mitchell, Daniela Negru, Charles and Lulu Nugent, Jim Pellmann, Jiří Pšenička, Jörn Rittweger, Valeriu

Rosetnic, Hilary Shirazi, Paul Sinton-Hewitt, Petr Soukup, Harmander Singh, Andrzej Szkandera, Ewa Urbańczyk-Piskorska, Andy Varns, Boff Whalley, Kirsty Woodbridge, Zygmund Worsa; and Zuzana Chmelová, J. Crowley and Ian Thompson. The last three, sadly, did not live to see this book published.

I have also benefited from the work of many authors and journalists who have covered these themes before me. There are, again, too many to list; but I acknowledge a particular debt to two excellent books: *What Makes Olga Run?* by Bruce Grierson; and *When Running Made History* by Roger Robinson.

I am also very grateful to my agent, Victoria Hobbs at A. H. Heath, for her unflappable support, and to Tim Broughton, Joe Pickering, Ellie Steel and Rhiannon Roy, who, at Yellow Jersey and Penguin Random House, have shepherded my book through the various stages of its long journey. And I am particularly grateful to Graham Coster, without whose inspired, patient and supportive editing this book would have been a lot longer, and considerably less coherent or readable, than it is. Its remaining shortcomings are all my own work.

Finally, I am grateful once again for the love and tolerance of my family: Clare; Isobel and Edward; and Anne and David. I am – as readers will already have gathered – unusually fortunate in many ways, without having done anything much to deserve it.

List of Illustrations

Ed Whitlock © Jim Ross / Toronto Star via Getty Images

Olga Kotelko © Alex Rotas

Earl Fee © Alex Rotas

Yoko Nakano © Robert Jerome

Stanislaw Kowalski (left) © Maciej Kulczynski/EPA/Shutterstock; Stanislaw Kowalski (right) © Richard Askwith

Ida Keeling © Poon Watchara-Amphaiwan

Elena Pagu © Valeriu Rosetnic

Octogenarian parkrun, Bushy Park © Carol Dickinson

Ginette Bedard © Don Emmert / AFP via Getty Images

Fauja Singh © Jayne Russell / Getty Images

Tommy Hughes © Malcolm McCausland

Alan Carter © Alex Rotas

Charles Allie © Alex Rotas

Angela Copson © Alex Rotas

Jo Pavey © Olivier Morin / AFP via Getty Images

Virginia Mitchell © Alex Rotas

penguin.co.uk/vintage